When

the

Body

Says

No

WHEN

THE

BODY

Exploring the
Stress-Disease Connection

SAYS NO

Gabor Maté, M.D.

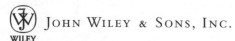
JOHN WILEY & SONS, INC.

Published by John Wiley & Sons, Inc., Hoboken, New Jersey

First published by Alfred A. Knopf in Canada in 2003

Page 296 constitutes a continuation of the copyright page.

For general information about our other products and services, please contact our
Customer Care Department within the United States at (800) 762-2974, outside the
United States at (317) 572-3993 or fax (317) 572-4002.

Wiley also publishes its books in a variety of electronic formats. Some content that appears in print may not be available in electronic books. For more information about Wiley
products, visit our web site at www.wiley.com.

ISBN 978-0-471-21982-8 (cloth); ISBN 978-0-470-92335-1 (pbk.); ISBN 978-1-118-
02787-5 (ebk); ISBN 978-0-471-46955-1 (ebk); ISBN 978-1-118-02510-9 (ebk);
ISBN 978-1-63026-256-3 (hc)

Printed in the United States of America

I dedicate this book to the memory of my mother, Judith Lövi, 1919–2001. And to the memory of Dr. Hans Selye, a twentieth-century Renaissance man whose scientific insights and humane wisdom continue to illuminate.

It is not to see something first, but to establish solid connections between the previously known and the hitherto unknown, that constitutes the essence of scientific discovery. It is this process of tying together which can best promote true understanding and real progress.

HANS SELYE, M.D., *The Stress of Life*

Contents

Preface

WHEN THE BODY SAYS NO has appeared in over fifteen languages on five continents. Its universal thesis is that mind and body are inseparable and that illness and health cannot be understood in isolation from the life histories, social context, and emotional patterns of human beings. Since the book's publication in 2003, much new information has accumulated to support this perspective.

A U.S. study, for example, found that women who are unhappily married and do not express their emotions have a greatly increased risk of death compared with similarly unhappy women who do not repress their feelings. Canadian research has shown that people abused in childhood have a nearly 50 percent increased risk of cancer in adulthood. Such data are manifestations of what the psychiatrist and author Daniel Siegel has termed "interpersonal neurobiology," or what, going a small step further, we may call *interpersonal biology*. Our relationships help shape our physiology.

As ancient philosophies and healing practices of cultures around the world have recognized, everything is interconnected. Despite breathtaking scientific advances in delineating that unity, we have not appreciated its implications and have not incorporated it into our medical practice. The war on cancer, for all its triumphs, has generally been a failure because it looks for the causes of malignancy in minute cellular mechanisms. As an astute observer has pointed out, attempting to find the cause of cancer on the cellular level is like trying to understand a traffic jam by examining the internal combustion engine. For the same reason, genomic research is also unable to illuminate the origins and treatment of illness.

This book shows that people do not become ill despite their lives but rather because of their lives. And life includes not only physical factors like diet, physical activity, and the environment, but also the internal milieu of thoughts and unconscious emotions that govern so much of our physiology, through the mechanisms of stress and the unity of the systems that modulate nerves, hormones, immunity, digestion, and cardiovascular function. Much disease could be prevented and healed if we fully understood the scientific evidence verifying the mind-body unity.

When the Body Says No is a not a book of prescriptions but rather one intended to encourage self-examination, insight, and transformation. As the great physiologist Walter Cannon suggested, there is an innate wisdom in our bodies. May we align with the inner wisdom we all possess.

Some of the case examples are derived from published biographies or autobiographies of well-known persons. The majority are taken from my clinical experience or from taped discussions with people who agreed to be interviewed and quoted regarding their medical and personal histories. For privacy reasons names (and, in some instances, other circumstances) have been changed.

To avoid making this work prohibitively academic for the lay reader, footnotes have been used only sparingly. References as well as an extensive bibliography are provided for each chapter at the end of the book. Italics, unless otherwise noted, are mine.

I welcome questions or comments at my Web site: www.drgabor mate.com.

1

The Bermuda Triangle

ARY WAS A NATIVE WOMAN in her early forties, slight of stature, gentle and deferential in manner. She had been my patient for eight years, along with her husband and three children. There was a shyness in her smile, a touch of self-deprecation. She laughed easily. When her ever-youthful face brightened, it was impossible not to respond in kind. My heart still warms—and constricts with sorrow—when I think of Mary.

Mary and I had never talked much until the illness that was to take her life gave its first signals. The beginning seemed innocent enough: a sewing-needle puncture wound on a fingertip failed over several months to heal. The problem was traced to Raynaud's phenomenon, in which the small arteries supplying the fingers are narrowed, depriving the tissues of oxygen. Gangrene can set in, and unfortunately this was the case for Mary. Despite several hospitalizations and surgical procedures, she was within a year begging for an amputation to rid her of the throbbing ache in her finger. By the time she got her wish the disease was rampant, and powerful narcotics were inadequate in the face of her constant pain.

Raynaud's can occur independently or in the wake of other disorders. Smokers are at greater risk, and Mary had been a heavy smoker since her teenage years. I hoped that if she quit, normal blood flow might return to her fingers. After many relapses she finally succeeded. Unfortunately, the Raynaud's proved to be the harbinger of something far worse: Mary was diagnosed with scleroderma, one of the autoimmune diseases, which include rheumatoid arthritis, ulcerative colitis, systemic lupus erythematosus (SLE) and many other conditions that are not always recognized to be autoimmune in origin, such as diabetes, multiple sclerosis and possibly even Alzheimer's disease. Common to them all is an attack by one's own immune system against the body, causing damage to joints, connective tissue or to almost any organ, whether it be the eyes, the nerves, the skin, the intestines, the liver or the brain. In scleroderma (from the Greek word meaning "hardened skin"), the immune system's suicidal assault results in a stiffening of the skin, esophagus, heart and tissues in the lungs and elsewhere.

What creates this civil war inside the body?

Medical textbooks take an exclusively biological view. In a few isolated cases, toxins are mentioned as causative factors, but for the most part a genetic predisposition is assumed to be largely responsible. Medical practice reflects this narrowly physical mindset. Neither the specialists nor I as her family doctor had ever thought to consider what in Mary's particular experiences might also have contributed to her illness. None of us expressed curiosity about her psychological state before the onset of the disease, or how this influenced its course and final outcome. We simply treated each of her physical symptoms as they presented themselves: medications for inflammation and pain, operations to remove gangrenous tissue and to improve blood supply, physiotherapy to restore mobility.

One day, almost on a whim, in response to a whisper of intuition that she needed to be heard, I invited Mary to make an hour-long appointment so that she would have the opportunity to tell me something about herself and her life. When she began to talk, it was a revelation. Beneath her meek and diffident manner was a vast store of repressed emotion. Mary had been abused as a child, abandoned and shuttled from one foster home to another. She recalled huddling in the attic at the age of seven, cradling her younger sisters in her arms, while her drunken foster parents fought and yelled below. "I was so scared all the time," she said, "but as a seven-year-old I had to protect my sisters. And no one protected me." She had never revealed these traumas before, not even to her husband of twenty years. She had learned not to express her feelings about anything to anyone, including herself. To be self-expressive, vulnerable and questioning in her childhood would have put her at risk. Her security lay in considering other people's feelings, never her own. She was trapped in the role forced on her as a child, unaware that she herself had the right to be taken care of, to be listened to, to be thought worthy of attention.

Mary described herself as being incapable of saying no, compulsively taking responsibility for the needs of others. Her major concern continued to be her husband and her nearly adult children, even as her illness became more grave. Was the scleroderma her body's way of finally rejecting this all-encompassing dutifulness?

Perhaps her body was doing what her mind could not: throwing off the relentless expectation that had been first imposed on the child and now was self-imposed in the adult—placing others above herself. I suggested as much when I wrote about Mary in my very first article as medical columnist for *The Globe and Mail* in 1993. "When we have been prevented from learning how to say no," I wrote, "our bodies may end up saying it for us." I cited some of the medical literature discussing the negative effects of stress on the immune system.

The idea that people's emotional coping style can be a factor in scleroderma or other chronic conditions is anathema to some physicians. A rheumatic diseases specialist at a major Canadian hospital submitted a scathing letter to the editor denouncing both my article and the newspaper for printing it. I was inexperienced, she charged, and had done no research.

That a specialist would dismiss the link between body and mind was not astonishing. Dualism—cleaving into two that which is one—colours all our beliefs on health and illness. We attempt to understand the body in isolation from the mind. We want to describe human beings—healthy or otherwise—as though they function in isolation from the environment in which they develop, live, work, play, love and die. These are the built-in, hidden biases of the medical orthodoxy that most physicians absorb during their training and carry into their practice.

Unlike many other disciplines, medicine has yet to assimilate an important lesson of Einstein's theory of relativity: that the position of an observer will influence the phenomenon being observed and affect the results of the observation. The unexamined assumptions of the scientist both determine and limit what he or she will discover, as the pioneering Czech-Canadian stress researcher Hans Selye pointed out. "Most people do not fully realize to what extent the spirit of scientific research and the lessons learned from it depend upon the personal viewpoints of the discoverers," he wrote in *The Stress of Life.* "In an age so largely dependent upon science and scientists, this fundamental point deserves special attention."[1] In that honest and self-revealing assessment Selye, himself a physician, expressed a truth that even now, a quarter century later, few people grasp.

The more specialized doctors become, the more they know about a body part or organ and the less they tend to understand the human being in whom that part or organ resides. The people I interviewed for this book reported nearly unanimously that neither their specialists nor their family doctors had ever invited them to explore the personal, subjective content of their lives. If anything, they felt that such a dialogue was discouraged in most of their contacts with the medical profession. In talking with my specialist colleagues about these very same patients, I found that even after many years of treating a person, a doctor could remain quite in the dark about the patient's life and experience outside the narrow boundaries of illness.

In this volume I set out to write about the effects of stress on health, particularly of the hidden stresses we all generate from our early programming, a pattern so deep and so subtle that it feels like a part of our real selves. Although I have presented as much of the available scientific evidence as seemed reasonable in a work for the lay public, the heart of the book—for me, at least—is formed by the individual histories I have been able to share with the readers. It so happens that those histories will also be seen as the least persuasive to those who regard such evidence as "anecdotal."

Only an intellectual Luddite would deny the enormous benefits that have accrued to humankind from the scrupulous application of scientific methods. But not all essential information can be confirmed in the laboratory or by statistical analysis. Not all aspects of illness can be reduced to facts verified by double-blind studies and by the strictest scientific techniques. "Medicine tells us as much about the meaningful performance of healing, suffering and dying as chemical analysis tells us about the aesthetic value of pottery," Ivan Ilyich wrote in *Limits to Medicine.* We confine ourselves to a narrow realm indeed if we exclude from accepted knowledge the contributions of human experience and insight.

We have lost something. In 1892 the Canadian William Osler, one of the greatest physicians of all time, suspected rheumatoid arthritis—a condition related to scleroderma—to be a stress-related disorder. Today rheumatology all but ignores that wisdom, despite the supporting scientific evidence accumulated in the 110 years since Osler first published his text. That is where the narrow scientific approach has brought the practice of medicine. In elevating modern science to be the final arbiter of our sufferings, we have been too eager to discard the insights of previous ages.

As the American psychologist Ross Buck has pointed out, until the advent of modern medical technology and of scientific pharmacology, physicians traditionally had to rely on "placebo" effects. They had to inspire in each patient a confidence in his, the patient's, inner ability to heal. To be effective, a doctor had to listen to the patient, to develop a relationship with him, and he had also to trust his own intuitions. Those are the qualities doctors seem to have lost as we have come to rely almost exclusively on "objective" measures, technology-based diagnostic methods and "scientific" cures.

Thus the rebuke from the rheumatologist was not a surprise. More of a jolt was another letter to the editor, a few days later—this time a supportive one—from Noel B. Hershfield, clinical professor of medicine at the University of Calgary: "The new discipline of psychoneuroimmunology has now matured to the point where there is compelling evidence, advanced by scientists from many fields, that an intimate relationship exists between the brain and the immune system. . . . An individual's emotional makeup, and the response to continued stress, may indeed be causative in the many diseases that medicine treats but whose [origin] is not yet known—diseases such as scleroderma, and the vast majority of rheumatic disorders, the inflammatory bowel disorders, diabetes, multiple sclerosis, and legions of other conditions which are represented in each medical subspecialty. . . ."

The surprising revelation in this letter was the existence of a new field of medicine. What is *psychoneuroimmunology*? As I learned, it is no less than the science of the interactions of mind and body, the indissoluble unity of emotions and physiology in human development and throughout life in health and illness. That dauntingly complicated word means simply that this discipline studies the ways that the psyche—the mind and its content of emotions—profoundly interacts with the body's nervous system and how both of them, in turn, form an essential link with our immune defences. Some have called this new field *psychoneuroimmunoendocrinology* to indicate that the endocrine, or hormonal, apparatus is also a part of our system of whole-body response. Innovative research is uncovering just how these links function all the way down to the cellular level. We are discovering the scientific basis of what we have known before and have forgotten, to our great loss.

Many doctors over the centuries came to understand that emotions are deeply implicated in the causation of illness or in the restoration of health. They did research, wrote books and challenged the reigning medical ideology, but repeatedly their ideas, explorations and insights vanished in a sort of medical Bermuda Triangle. The understanding of the mind–body connection achieved by previous generations of doctors and scientists disappeared without a trace, as if it had never seen daylight.

A 1985 editorial in the august *New England Journal of Medicine* could declare with magisterial self-assurance that "it is time to acknowledge that our belief in disease as a direct reflection of mental state is largely folklore."[2]

Such dismissals are no longer tenable. Psychoneuroimmunology, the new science Dr. Hershfield mentioned in his letter to the *The Globe and Mail,* has come into its own, even if its insights have yet to penetrate the world of medical practice.

A cursory visit to medical libraries or to online sites is enough to show the advancing tide of research papers, journal articles and textbooks discussing the new knowledge. Information has filtered down to many people in popular books and magazines. The lay public, ahead of the professionals in many ways and less shackled to old orthodoxies, finds it less threatening to accept that we cannot be divided up so easily and that the whole wondrous human organism is more than simply the sum of its parts.

Our immune system does not exist in isolation from daily experience. For example, the immune defences that normally function in healthy young people have been shown to be suppressed in medical students under the pressure of final examinations. Of even greater implication for their future health and well-being, the loneliest students suffered the greatest negative impact on their immune systems. Loneliness has been similarly associated with diminished immune activity in a group of psychiatric inpatients. Even if no further research evidence existed— though there is plenty—one would have to consider the long-term effects of chronic stress. The pressure of examinations is obvious and short term, but many people unwittingly spend their entire lives as if under the gaze of a powerful and judgmental examiner whom they must please at all costs. Many of us live, if not alone, then in emotionally inadequate relationships that do not recognize or honour our deepest needs. Isolation and stress affect many who may believe their lives are quite satisfactory.

How may stress be transmuted into illness? Stress is a complicated cascade of physical and biochemical responses to powerful emotional stimuli. Physiologically, emotions are themselves electrical, chemical and hormonal discharges of the human nervous system. Emotions influence—and are influenced by—the functioning of our major organs, the integrity of our immune defences and the workings of the many circulating biological substances that help govern the body's physical states. When emotions are repressed, as Mary had to do in her childhood search for security, this inhibition disarms the body's defences against illness. Repression—dissociating emotions from awareness and relegating them to the unconscious realm—disorganizes and confuses our physiological defences so that in some people these defences go awry, becoming the destroyers of health rather than its protectors.

During the seven years I was medical coordinator of the Palliative Care Unit at Vancouver Hospital, I saw many patients with chronic illness whose emotional histories resembled Mary's. Similar dynamics and ways of coping were present in the people who came to us for palliation with cancers or degenerative neurological processes like amyotrophic lateral sclerosis (ALS, also known in North America as Lou Gehrig's disease, after the great American baseball player who succumbed to it, and in Britain as motor neuron disease.) In my private family practice, I observed these same patterns in people I treated for multiple sclerosis, inflammatory ailments of the bowel such as ulcerative colitis and Crohn's disease, chronic fatigue syndrome, autoimmune disorders, fibromyalgia, migraine, skin disorders, endometriosis and many other conditions. In important areas of their lives, almost none of my patients with serious disease had ever learned to say no. If some people's personalities and circumstances appeared very different from Mary's on the surface, the underlying emotional repression was an ever-present factor.

One of the terminally ill patients under my care was a middle-aged man, chief executive of a company that marketed shark cartilage as a treatment for cancer. By the time he was admitted to our unit, his own recently diagnosed cancer had spread throughout his body. He continued to eat shark cartilage almost to the day of his death, but not because he any longer believed in its value. It smelled foul—the offensive stench was noticeable even some distance away—and I could only imagine what it tasted like. "I hate it," he told me, "but my business partner would be so disappointed if I stopped." I convinced him that he had every right to live his last days without feeling responsible for someone else's disappointment.

It is a sensitive matter to raise the possibility that the way people have been conditioned to live their lives may contribute to their illness. The connections between behaviour and subsequent disease are obvious in the case of, say, smoking and lung cancer—except perhaps to tobacco-industry executives. But such links are harder to prove when it comes to emotions and the emergence of multiple sclerosis or cancer of the breast or arthritis. In addition to being stricken with disease, the patient feels blamed for being the very person she is. "Why are you writing this book?" said a fifty-two-year-old university professor who has been treated for breast cancer. In a voice edged with anger she told me, "I got cancer because of my genes, not because of anything I did."

"The view of sickness and death as a personal failure is a particularly unfortunate form of blaming the victim," charged the 1985 editorial in the *New England Journal of Medicine*. "At a time when patients are already burdened by disease, they should not be further burdened by having to accept responsibility for the outcome."

We will return to this vexing question of assumed blame. Here I will only remark that blame and failure are not the issue. Such terms only cloud the picture. As we shall see, blaming the sufferer—apart from being morally obtuse—is completely unfounded from a scientific point of view.

The *NEJM* editorial confused blame and responsibility. While all of us dread being *blamed*, we all would wish to be more *responsible*—that is, to have the ability to *respond* with awareness to the circumstances of our lives rather than just reacting. We want to be the authoritative person in our own lives: in charge, able to make the authentic decisions that affect us. There is no true responsibility without awareness. One of the weaknesses of the Western medical approach is that we have made the physician the only authority, with the patient too often a mere recipient of the treatment or cure. People are deprived of the opportunity to become truly responsible. None of us are to be blamed if we succumb to illness and death. Any one of us might succumb at any time, but the more we can learn about ourselves, the less prone we are to become passive victims.

Mind and body links have to be seen not only for our understanding of illness but also for our understanding of health. Dr. Robert Maunder, on the psychiatric faculty of the University of Toronto, has written about the mind–body interface in disease. "Trying to identify and to answer the question of stress," he said to me in an interview, "is more likely to lead to health than ignoring the question." In healing, every bit of information, every piece of the truth, may be crucial. If a link exists between emotions and physiology, *not* to inform people of it will deprive them of a powerful tool.

And here we confront the inadequacy of language. Even to speak about links between mind and body is to imply that two discrete entities are somehow connected to each other. Yet in life there is no such separation; there is no body that is not mind, no mind that is not body. The word *mindbody* has been suggested to convey the real state of things.

Not even in the West is mind–body thinking completely new. In one of Plato's dialogues, Socrates quotes a Thracian doctor's criticism of his Greek colleagues: "This is the reason why the cure of so many diseases is unknown to the physicians of Hellas; they are ignorant of the whole. For this is the great error of our day in the treatment of the human body, that physicians separate the mind from the body."[3] You cannot split mind from body, said Socrates—nearly two and a half millennia before the advent of psychoneuroimmunoendocrinology!

Writing *When the Body Says No* has done more than simply confirm some of the insights I first articulated in my article about Mary's scleroderma. I have learned a great deal and have come to appreciate deeply the work of hundreds of physicians, scientists, psychologists and researchers who have charted the previously unmapped terrain of mind–body. Work on this book has also been an inner exploration of the ways I have repressed my own emotions. I was prompted to make this personal journey in response to a question from a counsellor at the British Columbia Cancer Agency, where I had gone to investigate the role of emotional repression in cancer. In many people with malignancy, there seemed to be an automatic denial of psychic or physical pain and of uncomfortable emotions like anger, sadness or rejection. "Just what is your personal connection to the issue?" the counsellor asked me. "What draws you to this particular topic?"

The question brought to mind an incident from seven years ago. One evening I arrived to see my seventy-six-year-old mother at the nursing home where she was a resident. She had progressive muscular dystrophy, an inherited muscle-wasting disease that runs in our family. Unable to even sit up without assistance, she could no longer live at home. Her three sons and their families visited her regularly until her death, which occurred just as I began to write this book.

I had a slight limp as I walked down the nursing home corridor. That morning I had undergone surgery for a torn cartilage in my knee, a consequence of ignoring what my body had been telling me in the language of pain that occurred each time I jogged on cement. As I opened the door to my mother's room, I automatically walked with a nonchalant, normal gait to her bed to greet her. The impulse to hide the limp was not conscious, and the act was done before I was aware of it. Only later did I wonder what exactly had prompted such an unnecessary measure—unnecessary because my mother would have calmly accepted that her fifty-one-year-old son would have a gimpy knee twelve hours post-surgery.

So what had happened? My automatic impulse to protect my mother from my pain, even in such an innocuous situation, was a deeply programmed reflex that had little to do with the present needs of either of us. That repression was a memory—a re-enactment of a dynamic that had been etched into my developing brain before I could possibly have been aware of it.

I am both a survivor and a child of the Nazi genocide, having lived most of my first year in Budapest under Nazi occupation. My maternal grandparents were killed in Auschwitz when I was five months old; my aunt had also been deported and was unheard from; and my father was in a forced labour battalion in the service of the German and Hungarian armies. My mother and I barely survived our months in the Budapest ghetto. For a few weeks she had to part from me as the only way of saving me from sure death by starvation or disease. No great powers of imagination are required to understand that in her state of mind, and under the inhuman stresses she was facing daily, my mother was rarely up to the tender smiles and undivided attention a developing infant requires to imprint a sense of security and unconditional love in his mind. My mother, in fact, told me that on many days her despair was such that only the need to care for me motivated her to get up from bed. I learned early that I had to work for attention, to burden my mother as little as possible and that my anxiety and pain were best suppressed.

In healthy mother–infant interactions, the mother is able to nourish without the infant's having in any way to work for what he receives. My mother was unable to provide that unconditional nourishing for me—and since she was neither saintly nor perfect, quite likely she would not have completely succeeded in doing so, even without the horrors that beset our family.

It was under these circumstances that I became my mother's protector—protecting her in the first instance against awareness of my own pain. What began as the automatic defensive coping of the infant soon hardened into a fixed personality pattern that, fifty-one years later, still caused me to hide even my slightest physical discomfort in front of my mother.

I had not thought about the *When the Body Says No* project in those terms. This was to be an intellectual quest, to explore an interesting theory that would help explain human health and illness. It was a path others had trod before me, but there was always more to be discovered. The counsellor's challenge made me confront the issue of emotional repression in my own life. My hidden limp, I realized, was only one small example.

Thus, in writing this book, I describe not only what I have learned from others or from professional journals but also what I have observed in myself. The dynamics of repression operate in all of us. We are all self-deniers and self-betrayers to one extent or another, most often in ways we are no more aware of than I was conscious of while "deciding" to disguise my limp. When it comes to health or illness, it is only a matter of degree and, too, a matter of the presence or absence of other factors—such as heredity or environmental hazards, for example—that also predispose to disease. So in demonstrating that repression is a major cause of stress and a significant contributor to illness, I do not point fingers at others for "making themselves sick." My purpose in this book is to promote learning and healing, not to add to the quotient of blame and shame, both of which already exist in overabundance in our culture. Perhaps I am overly sensitized to the issue of blame, but then most people are. Shame is the deepest of the "negative emotions," a feeling we will do almost anything to avoid. Unfortunately, our abiding fear of shame impairs our ability to see reality.

Despite the best efforts of many physicians, Mary died in Vancouver Hospital eight years after her diagnosis, succumbing to the complications of scleroderma. To the end she retained her gentle smile, though her heart was weak and her breathing laboured. Every once in a while she would ask me to schedule long private visits, even in hospital during her final days. She just wanted to chat, about matters serious or trivial. "You are the only one who ever listened to me," she once said.

I have wondered at times how Mary's life might have turned out if someone had been there to hear, see and understand her when she was a small child—abused, frightened, feeling responsible for her little sisters. Perhaps had someone been there consistently and dependably, she could have learned to value herself, to express her feelings, to assert her anger when people invaded her boundaries physically or emotionally. Had that been her fate, would she still be alive?

2

The Little Girl Too Good

to Be True

T WOULD BE AN UNDERSTATEMENT to say that the spring and summer of 1996 was a stressful time in Natalie's life. In March her sixteen-year-old son was discharged from a six-month stay at a drug rehabilitation facility. He had used drugs and alcohol for the previous two years and was repeatedly expelled from school. "We were lucky we got him into the residential treatment program," says the fifty-three-year-old former nurse. "He had only been home a short while when first my husband was diagnosed, and then me." In July her husband, Bill, underwent surgery for a malignant bowel tumour. After the operation they were told the cancer had spread to his liver.

Natalie had suffered fatigue, dizziness and ringing in her ears from time to time, but her symptoms were of short duration and resolved without treatment. In the year before her diagnosis she had felt more tired than usual. A bout of vertigo in June led to a CT scan, with negative results. Two months later an MRI of Natalie's brain showed the characteristic abnormalities associated with multiple sclerosis: focal areas of inflammation where myelin, the fatty tissue lining nerve cells, was damaged and scarred.

Multiple sclerosis (from the Greek, "to harden") is the most common of the so-called demyelinating diseases that impair the functioning of cells in the central nervous system. Its symptoms depend on where the inflammation and scarring occur. The main areas attacked are usually the spinal cord, the brain stem and the optic nerve, which is the bundle of nerve fibres carrying visual information to the brain. If the site of damage is somewhere in the spinal cord, the symptoms will be numbness, pain or other unpleasant sensations in the limbs or trunk. There may also be involuntary tightening of the muscles or weakness. In the lower part of the brain, the loss of myelin can induce double vision or problems with speech or balance. Patients with optic neuritis—inflammation of the optic nerve—suffer temporary visual loss. Fatigue is a common symptom, a sense of overwhelming exhaustion far beyond ordinary tiredness.

Natalie's dizziness continued through the fall and early winter while she nursed her husband through his convalescence from the bowel operation and a twelve-week course of chemotherapy. For a while afterwards Bill was able to resume his work as a real estate agent. Then in May 1997 a second operation was performed to excise the tumours in his liver.

"Following the resection, in which they removed 75 per cent of his liver, Bill developed a blood clot in his portal vein.* He could have died from that," says Natalie. "He became very confused and combative." Bill died in 1999, but not before subjecting his wife to more emotional agony than she could have foreseen.

Researchers in Colorado looked at one hundred people with the type of MS called relapsing-remitting, in which flare-ups alternate with symptom-free periods. This is the type Natalie has. Patients burdened by qualitatively extreme stresses, such as major relationship difficulties or financial insecurity, were almost four times as likely to suffer exacerbations.[1]

"I was still having a lot of vertigo over Christmas of 1996, but after that I was almost 100 per cent," Natalie reports. "Only my gait was a little off. And despite all the problems with Bill's liver resection—I had to take him to the emergency ward four times between July and August—I was fine. It appeared Bill was turning around, and we were hopeful there would be no more complications. Then I had another exacerbation." The flare-up came when Natalie thought she could relax a little, when her services were no longer urgently needed.

---

* *The portal vein is the major vessel conveying blood from abdominal organs to the liver.*

"My husband was the type of person who felt that he shouldn't have to do anything he didn't want to do. He was always like that. When he was sick, he just figured he was definitely not going to do anything. He would sit down on the sofa and snap his fingers—and when he snapped, you jumped. Even the kids were getting very impatient with him. Finally, in the fall, when he was better, I sent him out of town for a few days with some friends. I said, 'He needs to get out.'"

"What did *you* need?" I ask.

"I was fed up. I said, 'Take him away to play some golf for a few days,' and this friend came and picked him up. And two hours later I knew I was having an exacerbation."

What might she have learned from this experience? "Well," Natalie says hesitantly, "that I need to know when to withdraw from my helping mode. But I just can't; if somebody needs help, I have to do it."

"Regardless of what's happening for you?"

"Yes. Five years down the road, and I still have not learned that I have to pace myself. My body says no to me frequently, and I keep going. I don't learn."

Natalie's body had many reasons to say no throughout her marriage. Bill was a heavy drinker and often embarrassed her. "When he would have a little too much to drink, he became ugly," she says. "He would be argumentative, aggressive, lose his temper. We would be out at a party, and if something upset him, he would tear strips off people in public, for no reason. I would just turn around and walk away, and then he would be angry with me for not supporting him. I knew within forty-eight hours of being diagnosed with MS that Bill would not be there for me."

Returning from his golfing vacation, Bill experienced some months of physical vigour. He engaged in a relationship with another woman, a friend of the family. "I thought, Look what I've done for you," says Natalie. "I've jeopardized my own health. I was there for you all summer. You were at death's door, and I sat for seventy-two hours in that hospital waiting to see if you were going to die or recover. I looked after you when you came home, and this is how I get paid back. I get kicked in the teeth."

The idea that psychological stress increases the risk for multiple sclerosis is not new. The French neurologist Jean-Martin Charcot was first to give a full clinical description of multiple sclerosis. Patients, he

reported in a lecture in 1868, connect "long continued grief or vexa-
tion" with the onset of symptoms. Five years later a British physician
described a case also associated with stress:"Aetiologically it is important
to mention another statement the poor creature made when giving a
more confidential account to the nurse—that the cause of her disease
was having caught her husband in bed with another woman."[2]

For this book I interviewed nine people with MS, eight of them
women. (About 60 per cent of those affected are women.) The emotional patterns illustrated in Natalie's story are evident in each person,
if not always as dramatically.

The evidence gathered from my interviews is consistent with the
published research. "Many students of this disease have voiced the clinical impression that emotional stress may be somehow implicated in the
genesis of MS," a research article noted in 1970.[3] Excessive emotional
involvement with a parent, a lack of psychological independence, an
overwhelming need for love and affection, and the inability to feel or
express anger have long been identified by medical observers as possible factors in the natural development of the disease. A study in 1958
found that in nearly 90 per cent of cases,"before the onset of symptoms
. . . patients experienced traumatic life events that had threatened their
'security system.'"[4]

A study done in 1969 looked at the role of psychological processes in
thirty-two patients from Israel and the United States. Eighty-five per cent
of these MS patients experienced the emergence of symptoms that were
subsequently diagnosed as multiple sclerosis in the wake of recent highly
stressful events. The nature of the stressor varied considerably, from the
death or illness of loved ones to a sudden threat of loss of livelihood or
perhaps to a family event that caused permanent change in a person's
life and demanded a flexibility or adaptation beyond his ability to manage. Protracted marital conflict was one such source of stress, increased
responsibility at work another. "The common characteristic . . ." write
the authors of the study, "is the gradual realization of the inability to
cope with a difficult situation . . . provoking feelings of inadequacy or
failure."[5] These stresses held across different cultures.

Another study compared MS patients with a group of healthy
"controls." Severely threatening events were ten times more common,
and marital conflict five times more frequent, in the MS group.[6]

Of the eight women with multiple sclerosis I spoke with, only one was still in her first long-term relationship; the others had separated or divorced. Four of the women had been abused physically or psychologically by their partners sometime before the onset of illness. In the remaining cases their partners had been emotionally distant and unavailable.

Lois, a journalist, was twenty-four when she was diagnosed with MS in 1974. A brief episode of double vision was followed some months later by pins-and-needles sensations in her legs. She had lived the previous two years in a small Native settlement in the Arctic with a man nine years her senior, an artist whom she now describes as mentally unstable. Later he was hospitalized for manic-depressive illness. "I idolized him," she recalls. "He was very talented, and I felt I didn't know anything. Maybe I was a little afraid of him."

Lois found life in the Arctic extremely difficult. "For a sheltered West Coast girl, it was like moving to Timbuctoo. I saw a psychologist years afterwards, and he said, 'You were lucky to get out of there alive.' There was a lot of drinking, death and murder, isolation. There's no road in there. I was physically afraid of my partner, of his judgment and his anger. It was a summer romance that should have lasted a few months, but it lasted a couple of years. I tried to hang on as hard as I could, but eventually he kicked me out."

The living conditions were bad. "We had an outhouse, and in −40 or −50 degree weather, that's awful. Then he conceded and got a honey bucket, as they called it, that I could pee into at night because women have to pee more than men, right?"

"That was a concession?" I inquire.

"Yes, right. We had to cart it away to dump it, and he didn't want to do that. One night he chucked it out in the snow and told me to use the outhouse. I also had to carry the water—we had no running water. There was no option. If I wanted to stay with him, I had to put up with that.

"I remember saying the main thing I wanted from him was respect. I don't know why, but that was the big thing for me. I wanted that so badly I was willing to put up with a lot."

Lois says that a desperate need for approval had characterized her earlier life as well, especially her relationship with her mother. "I transferred to him my mother always being in control of my life . . . telling me what to wear and decorating my room and telling me what I should do from the beginning. I was the little girl too good to be true. It means that you subjugate your own wants or needs in order to get approval. I was always trying to be who my parents wanted me to be."

Barbara, a psychotherapist—by reputation, a highly effective one—treats many people with chronic illness. She herself has multiple sclerosis. She strenuously objects to the suggestion that repression originating in her childhood experience has anything to do with the plaques of inflammation and scarring at the root of her MS symptoms.

Barbara's multiple sclerosis presented eighteen years ago. The first symptoms erupted shortly after she invited a sociopathic man she had worked with at a correctional facility into her home for a two-week stay. "He had done a lot of therapy," she says, "and the idea was to give him a fresh chance." Instead, the client caused havoc and disruption in her home and her marriage. I ask Barbara if she does not see this invitation to a seriously troubled person as having represented a major boundary problem on her part.

"Well, yes and no. I thought it was fine, because it was a two-week deal. But I would never do it again, obviously. I'm so good on boundaries now that I have one client who calls me the boundary queen—and she is another therapist, so we joke about it. Unfortunately, I had to learn the hard way. Sometimes I think that my MS was a punishment for my foolishness."

This reference to disease as punishment raises a key issue, since people with chronic illness are frequently accused, or may accuse themselves, of somehow deserving their misfortune. If the repression/stress perspective truly did imply that disease was punishment, I would agree with Barbara's rejection of it. But a search for scientific understanding is incompatible with moralizing and judgment. To say that an ill-advised decision to invite a potentially harmful person into one's home was a source of stress and played a role in the onset of illness is simply to point out a relationship between stress and disease. It is to discuss a possible consequence—not as punishment but as physiological reality.

Barbara insists she had nothing but a mutually loving and healthy relationship with her parents. "My mother and I were great together. We were always very close."

"Boundaries are learned in our formative years," I say. "So why did you have to learn boundaries later, the hard way?"

"I knew boundaries, but my mother did not. That's what most of our fights were about—about her inability to recognize where she ended and I began."

Barbara's introduction of an unstable and dangerous man into her home would be defined in studies as a major stressor, but the chronic stress of poor boundaries that preceded it is not so easily identified. The blurring of psychological boundaries during childhood becomes a significant source of future physiological stress in the adult. There are ongoing negative effects on the body's hormonal and immune systems, since people with indistinct personal boundaries live with stress; it is a permanent part of their daily experience to be encroached upon by others. However, that is a reality they have learned to exclude from direct awareness.

"The cause, or causes, of multiple sclerosis remain unknown," notes a respected textbook of internal medicine.[7] Most research refutes a contagious origin, although a virus may possibly be indicated. There are probably genetic influences, since a few racial groups do seem to be free of it—for example, the Inuit in North America and the Bantus of southern Africa. But genes do not explain who gets the disease or why. "While it is possible to inherit a genetic susceptibility to MS, *it is not possible to inherit the disease,*" writes the neurologist Louis J. Rosner, former head of the UCLA Multiple Sclerosis Clinic. "And even people who have all the necessary genes do not necessarily get MS. The disease, experts believe, must be triggered by environmental factors."[8]

Complicating matters are MRI studies and autopsies that identify the characteristic signs of demyelination in the central nervous system of persons who never exhibited any overt signs or symptoms of the disease. Why is it that some people with these neuropathological findings escape the frank development of illness while others do not?

What could be the "environmental factors" alluded to by Dr. Rosner?

Dr. Rosner's otherwise excellent primer on multiple sclerosis summarily dismisses exploration of emotional stress as contributing factor to the onset. Instead, he concludes that the disease is probably best explained by autoimmunity. "A person becomes allergic to his own tissue," he explains, "and produces antibodies that attack healthy cells." He ignores the abundant medical literature linking autoimmune processes themselves to stress and personality, a vital link to be explored more fully in later chapters.

A 1994 study done in the Department of Neurology at the University of Chicago Hospital looked at nervous system–immune system interactions and their potential role in multiple sclerosis.[9] Rats were used to demonstrate that artificially induced autoimmune disease would worsen when the flight-or-fight response was blocked. Had it not been interfered with, the animals' ability to respond normally to stress would have protected them.

The MS patients described in the stress literature, and all the ones I interviewed, have been placed in positions akin to that of the unfortunate laboratory animals in the Chicago study: they were exposed to acute and chronic stress by their childhood conditioning, and their ability to engage in the necessary flight-or-fight behaviour was impaired. The fundamental problem is not the external stress, such as the life events quoted in the studies, but an environmentally conditioned helplessness that permits neither of the normal responses of fight or flight. The resulting internal stress becomes repressed and therefore invisible. Eventually, having unmet needs or having to meet the needs of others is no longer experienced as stressful. It feels normal. One is disarmed.

Véronique is thirty-three; she was diagnosed with MS three years ago. "I had a major episode," she relates, "which I didn't know was an episode . . . pain in my feet, numbness and tingling going all the way up to about the upper chest and then back down, over about three days. I thought it was cool—I was poking myself and couldn't feel anything! I didn't say anything to anybody." A friend finally convinced her to seek medical help.

"You had numbness and pain from your feet to your upper chest and you didn't tell anybody? Why is that?"

"I didn't think it was worth telling anybody. And if I told somebody like my parents, they would be upset."

"But if someone else had numbness and pain from the feet up to the mid-chest, would you ignore it?"

"No, I would rush him to the doctor."

"Why were you treating yourself worse than you would another person? Any idea?"

"No."

Most instructive is Véronique's response to the question about any possibly stressful experiences prior to the onset of her multiple sclerosis. "Not necessarily bad things," she says.

"I'm an adopted child. Finally, after fifteen years of pressure from my adoptive mom, I looked up my biological family, which I didn't want to do. But it's always easier to give in to my mom's demands than argue about it—always!

"I found them and met them, and my very first impression was, Ugh, we can't possibly be related. It was stressful for me to find out about my family history because I didn't need to know that I was possibly a child of incestuous rape. That's how it appears; nobody's telling the whole story, and my biological mother won't say anything.

"Also at that time I was unemployed, waiting for EI, on welfare. And I'd kicked out my boyfriend a few months before this, because he was an alcoholic and I couldn't handle that any more either. It wasn't worth my sanity."

Such are the stresses this young woman describes as not necessarily bad: ongoing pressure from her adoptive mother, who ignored Véronique's own wishes, to find and reunite with her dysfunctional biological family; discovering that her conception may have been the result of incestuous rape (by a cousin; Véronique's biological mother was sixteen at the time); financial destitution; her break with an alcoholic boyfriend.

Véronique identifies with her adoptive father. "He's my hero," she says. "He was always there for me."

"So why didn't you go to him for help when you felt pressured by your mother?"

"I could never get him alone. I always had to go through her to get to him."

"And what did your father do with all this?"

"He just stood by. But I could tell he didn't like it."

"I'm glad you feel close to your dad. But you may wish to find yourself a new hero—one who can model some self-assertion. In order to heal, you may wish to become your own hero."

———

The gifted British cellist Jacqueline du Pré died in 1987, at the age of forty-two, from complications of multiple sclerosis. When her sister, Hilary, wondered later whether stress might have brought on Jackie's illness, the neurologists firmly assured her that stress was not implicated.

Orthodox medical opinion has shifted very little since then. "Stress does not cause multiple sclerosis," a pamphlet recently issued by the University of Toronto's MS clinic advised patients, "although people with MS are well advised to avoid stress." The statement is misleading. Of course stress does not *cause* multiple sclerosis—no single factor does. The emergence of MS no doubt depends on a number of interacting influences. But is it true to say that stress does not make a major contribution to the onset of this disease? Research studies and the lives of the persons we have looked at strongly suggest that it does. Such also is the evidence of the life Jacqueline du Pré, whose illness and death are a virtual textbook illustration of the devastating effects of the stress brought on by emotional repression.

People often wept at du Pre's concerts. Her communication with audiences, someone remarked, "was quite breathtaking and left everyone spellbound." Her playing was passionate, sometimes unbearably intense. She blazed a direct path to the emotions. Unlike her private persona, her stage presence was completely uninhibited: hair flying, body swaying, it was more typical of rock 'n' roll flamboyance than of classical restraint. "She appeared to be a sweet, demure milkmaid," an observer recalled, "but with cello in hands she was like one possessed."[10]

To this day some of du Pré's recorded performances, notably of the Elgar cello concerto, are unsurpassed—and are likely to remain so. This concerto was the eminent composer's last major work, created in a mood of despondency in the wake of the First World War. "Everything good and nice and clean and fresh and sweet is far away, never to return," Edward Elgar wrote in 1917. He was in his seventh decade, in the twilight of his years. "Jackie's ability to portray the emotions of a man in the autumn of his life was one of her extraordinary and inexplicable capacities," writes her sister, Hilary du Pré, in her book, *A Genius in the Family*.[11]

Extraordinary, yes. Inexplicable? Perhaps not. Although she was unaware of it, by the time she was twenty, Jacqueline du Pré was also in the autumn of her life. The illness that was soon to end her musical career was only a few years away. Regret, loss and resignation had all been too abundantly a part of her unspoken emotional experience. She understood Elgar because she had partaken of the same suffering. His portrait always disturbed her. "He had a miserable life, Hil," she told her sibling, "and he was ill, yet through it all he had a radiant soul, and that's what I feel in his music."

She was describing herself, from her earliest beginnings. Jackie's mother, Iris, suffered the death of her own father while she was still in the maternity hospital with Jackie. From then on, Jackie's relationship with her mother became one of symbiotic dependence from which neither party could free herself. The child was neither allowed to be a child nor permitted to grow up to be an adult.

Jackie was a sensitive child, quiet and shy, sometimes mischievous. She was said to have been placid, except when playing the cello. A music teacher recalls her at age six as having been "terribly polite and nicely brought up." She presented a pleasant and compliant face to the world. The secretary at the girls' school Jackie attended remembers her as a happy and cheerful child. A high-school classmate recalls her as a "friendly, jolly girl who fitted in well."

Jackie's inner reality was quite different. Hilary recounts that her sister burst into tears one day: "No one likes me at school. It's horrible. They all tease me." In an interview Jacqueline portrayed herself as "one of those children other children can't stand. They used to form gangs and chant horrid things." She was an awkward youngster, socially gauche, with no academic interests and little to say. According to her sister, Jackie always had difficulty expressing herself in words. "Observant friends noted an incipient strain of melancholy underneath Jackie's sunny exterior," writes her biographer, Elizabeth Wilson, in *Jacqueline du Pré*.[12]

All her life, until her illness, Jackie would hide her feelings from her mother. Hilary recalls a chilling childhood memory of Jacqueline's intense expression and secretive whisper, "Hil, don't tell Mum but . . . when I grow up, I won't be able to walk or move." How are we to understand that horrific self-prophecy? Either as something uncanny or as the projection of exactly how, in her unconscious depths, the child Jackie already felt: incapable of moving independently, fettered, her vital self paralyzed. And "don't tell Mum"? The resignation of someone already aware of the futility of trying to convey her pain, fear and anxiety—her shadow side—to a parent unable to receive such communication. Much later, when multiple sclerosis struck, all Jackie's lifelong resentment toward her mother erupted in bursts of uncontrolled, profane rage. The docile child became a profoundly hostile adult.

As much as Jacqueline du Pré loved and craved the cello, something in her resisted the role of cello virtuoso. This virtuoso persona pre-empted her true self. It also became her only mode of emotional communication and her only way of keeping her mother's attention. Multiple sclerosis was to be her means of casting off this role—her body's way of saying no.

Jacqueline herself was incapable of refusing the world's expectations directly. At the age of eighteen, already in the public eye, she was wistfully envious of another young cellist who was then experiencing a crisis. "That girl is lucky," she told a friend. "She could give up music if she wanted to. But I could never give it up because too many people have spent too much money on me." The cello enabled her to soar to unimaginable heights and it shackled her. Terrified as she was of the toll a musical career would take on her, she succumbed to the impositions of her talent and her family's needs.

Hilary speaks of Jackie's "cello voice." Because Jackie's direct means of emotional expression had been stifled early on, the cello became her voice. She poured all her intensity, pain, resignation—all her rage—into her music. As one of her cello teachers astutely observed when Jackie was an adolescent, she was forcing the instrument to express her internal aggression through her playing. When engaged in music, she was fully animated by emotions that were diluted or absent everywhere else in her life. This is why she was so was riveting to watch and so often painful to listen to—"almost scary" in the words of the Russian cellist Misha Maisky.

Twenty years after her childhood debut, now ill with MS, Jackie told a friend what she had felt on first finding herself on stage. "It was as if until that moment she had in front of her a brick wall which blocked her communication with the outside world. But the moment Jackie started to play for an audience, that brick wall vanished and she felt able to speak at last. It was a sensation that never left her when she performed." As an adult she was to write in her diary that she had never known how to speak in words, only through music.

Her relationship with her husband, Daniel Barenboim, dominated the last phase of Jacqueline du Pré's life before multiple sclerosis ended her cello playing. A charming, cultured and cosmopolitan Argentine Jew who had grown up in Israel, Barenboim by his early twenties was a supernova in the international musical galaxy. He was a sought-after concert pianist and chamber musician and was also making a name for himself as a conductor. When du Pré and Barenboim met, the musical communication between them was spontaneously electric, passionate, even mystical. A love affair and marriage were inevitable. It seemed a fairy-tale romance; they became the glamour couple of the classical music world.

Unfortunately, Jackie could no more be her true self in her marriage than in her family of origin. People who knew her well soon noticed that she spoke with a curious, "indefinable" mid-Atlantic accent. This unconscious adoption of her husband's mode of speaking signalled the merging of her identity with that of another, more dominant personality. Hilary writes that once more Jackie was fitting herself to someone else's needs and expectations: "The wide-open spaces of her personality had little chance for expression except through their music-making. *She had to be the Jackie the circumstances demanded.*"

When her yet-undiagnosed progressive neurological disease began to cause serious symptoms like weakness and falling, she followed a lifelong pattern of silence. Rather than alarm her husband, she hid her problems, pretending that other causes had slowed her down.

"Well, I can only say that it doesn't feel like stress," Jackie said one time, early in her marriage, when Hilary asked how she coped with the strain of both a personal and professional relationship with her husband. "I find myself a very happy person. I love my music and I love my husband and there seems to be ample time for both." A short while later she fled husband and career. She came to believe that her husband stood between her and her true self. She briefly left the marriage, acting out her unhappiness through a sexual affair with her brother-in-law—a further example of her uncertain boundaries. Deeply depressed, for a while she wanted nothing to do with the cello. Soon after she returned to both marriage and music, she was diagnosed with MS.

Jacqueline du Pré's cello voice remained her only voice. Hilary called it her sister's salvation. It was not. It worked for audiences, but it did not work for her. People loved her impassioned music making, but no one who mattered ever truly listened. Audiences wept and critics sang her praises, but no one heard her. Tragically, she, too, was deaf to her true self. Artistic expression by itself is only a form of acting out emotions, not a way of working them through.

After her sister's death, Hilary listened to a 1973 BBC tape of the Elgar concerto, with Zubin Mehta conducting. It had been Jackie's final public performance in Britain. "A few moments of tuning, a short pause, and she began. I suddenly jumped. She was slowing the tempo down. A few more bars and it became vividly clear. I knew exactly what was happening. Jackie, as always, was speaking through her cello. I could hear what she was saying. . . . I could almost see tears on her face. She was saying goodbye to herself, playing her own requiem."

3

Stress and

Emotional Competence

A PERENNIAL GIVE-AND-TAKE HAS been going on between living matter and its inanimate surroundings, between one living being and another, ever since the dawn of life in the prehistoric oceans," wrote Hans Selye in *The Stress of Life*.[1] Interactions with other human beings—in particular, emotional interactions—affect our biological functioning in myriad and subtle ways almost every moment of our lives. They are important determinants of health, as we will see throughout this book. Understanding the intricate balance of relationships among our psychological dynamics, our emotional environment and our physiology is crucial to well-being. "This may seem odd," wrote Selye. "You may feel that there is no conceivable relationship between the behaviour of our cells, for instance in inflammation, and our conduct in everyday life. I do not agree."[2]

Despite the intervening six decades of scientific inquiry since Selye's groundbreaking work, the physiological impact of the emotions is still far from fully appreciated. The medical approach to health and illness continues to suppose that body and mind are separable from each other and from the milieu in which they exist. Compounding that mistake is a definition of stress that is narrow and simplistic.

Medical thinking usually sees stress as highly disturbing but isolated events such as, for example, sudden unemployment, a marriage breakup or the death of a loved one. These major events are potent sources of stress for many, but there are chronic daily stresses in people's lives that are more insidious and more harmful in their long-term biological consequences. Internally generated stresses take their toll without in any way seeming out of the ordinary.

For those habituated to high levels of internal stress since early childhood, it is the absence of stress that creates unease, evoking boredom and a sense of meaninglessness. People may become addicted to their own stress hormones, adrenaline and cortisol, Hans Selye observed. To such persons stress feels desirable, while the absence of it feels like something to be avoided.

When people describe themselves as being stressed, they usually mean the nervous agitation they experience under excessive demands—most commonly in the areas of work, family, relationships, finances or health. But sensations of nervous tension do not define stress—nor, strictly speaking, are they always perceived when people are stressed. Stress, as we will define it, is not a matter of subjective feeling. It is a measurable set of objective physiological events in the body, involving the brain, the hormonal apparatus, the immune system and many other organs. Both animals and people can experience stress with no awareness of its presence.

"Stress is not simply nervous tension," Selye pointed out. "Stress reactions do occur in lower animals, and even in plants, that have no nervous systems. . . . Indeed, stress can be produced under deep anaesthesia in patients who are unconscious, and even in cell cultures grown outside the body."[3] Similarly, stress effects can be highly active in persons who are fully awake, but who are in the grip of unconscious emotions or cut off from their body responses. The physiology of stress may be triggered without observable effects on behaviour and without subjective awareness, as has been shown in animal experiments and in human studies.

What, then, is stress? Selye—who coined the word in its present usage and who described with mock pride how *der stress, le stress* and *lo stress* entered the German, French and Italian languages respectively—conceived of stress as a biological process, a wide-ranging set of events in the body, irrespective of cause or of subjective awareness. Stress consists of the internal alterations—visible or not—that occur when the organism perceives a threat to its existence or well-being. While nervous tension may be a component of stress, one can be stressed without feeling tension. On the other hand, it is possible to feel tension without activating the physiological mechanisms of stress.

In searching for a word to capture the meaning of the physical changes he observed in his experiments, Selye "stumbled upon the term *stress*, which had long been used in common English, and particularly in engineering, to denote the effects of a force acting against a resistance." He gives the example of changes induced in a stretched rubber band or in a steel spring under pressure. These changes may be noted with the naked eye or may be evident only on microscopic examination.

Selye's analogies illustrate an important point: excessive stress occurs when the demands made on an organism exceed that organism's reasonable capacities to fulfill them. The rubber band snaps, the spring becomes deformed. The stress response can be set off by physical damage, either by infection or injury. It can also be triggered by emotional trauma or just by the threat of such trauma, even if purely imaginary. Physiological stress responses can be evoked when the threat is outside conscious awareness or even when the individual may believe himself to be stressed in a "good" way.

Alan, a forty-seven-year-old engineer, was diagnosed with cancer of the esophagus—the swallowing tube that carries food from the throat to the stomach—a few years ago. He spoke of "good stress" when he described the relentless, self-driven existence he had led in the year before he was diagnosed with his malignancy. That "good stress" not only helped undermine his health, but it also served to distract him from painful issues in his life that were themselves constant sources of ongoing physiological disturbance in his system.

Alan's lower esophagus has been removed, along with the upper portion of the stomach where the tumour had invaded. Because the cancer had spread to several lymph nodes outside the gut, he received five courses of chemotherapy. His white blood cells became so depleted that another round of chemo would have killed him.

A non-smoker or drinker, he was shocked by the diagnosis, since he always considered that he lived a healthy life. But he has thought for a long time that he has a "weak stomach." He often suffered indigestion and heartburn, a symptom of the reflux of stomach acid into the esophagus.

The lining of the esophagus is not designed to withstand the corrosive bath of hydrochloric acid secreted in the stomach. A muscular valve between the two organs and complex neurological mechanisms ensure that food can move downward from throat to stomach without permitting acid to flow back upward. Chronic reflux can damage the surface of the lower esophagus, predisposing it to malignant change.

Not being one to complain, Alan had only once mentioned this problem to doctors. He thinks fast, speaks fast, does everything fast. He believed, quite plausibly, in fact, that his habit of eating on the run was responsible for the heartburn. However, excessive acid production due to stress and disordered neural input from the autonomic nervous system also play a role in reflux. The autonomic part of the nervous system is the part not under our conscious control, and—as the name implies—it is responsible for many automatic body functions such as heart rate, breathing and the muscle contractions of internal organs.

I asked Alan if there had been any stresses in his life in the period preceding the diagnosis. "Yes. I had been under stress, but there are two kinds of stress. There is stress that is bad and stress that is good." In Alan's estimation the "bad stress" was the complete lack of intimacy in his ten-year marriage to Shelley. He sees that as the main reason the couple have not had children. "She just has some very serious problems. Because of her inability to be romantic, intimate and all the things that I need, my frustrations with our marriage were at their absolute peak at the point I got the cancer. I've always felt that that was a really major thing." The "good stresses," in Alan's view, came from his work. In the year prior to his diagnosis he worked eleven hours a day, seven days a week. I asked him if he has ever said no to anything.

"Never. In fact, I love being asked. Almost never have I said yes with deep regret. I like doing things, I like taking things on. All somebody has to do is ask me and they got me."

"What about since the cancer?"

"I've learned to say no—I say it all the time. I want to live! I think saying no plays a big role in getting better. Four years ago they gave me a 15 per cent chance of survival. I made a conscious decision that I wanted to live, and I set a timeline somewhere between five and seven years.

"How do you mean?"

"Five years is supposed to be the magical thing, but I know it's just an arbitrary timeline. I figure I'll cheat and get two more years. Then, after seven . . ."

"Are you saying that after seven years you can go back to living crazily again?"

"Yes, I might. I don't know."

"Big mistake!"

"Probably—we'll talk about that. But right now I'm a good boy. I really am. I say no to everybody."

The experience of stress has three components. The first is the event, physical or emotional, that the organism interprets as threatening. This is the stress stimulus, also called the *stressor.* The second element is the processing system that experiences and interprets the meaning of the stressor. In the case of human beings, this processing system is the nervous system, in particular the brain. The final constituent is the stress response, which consists of the various physiological and behavioural adjustments made as a reaction to a perceived threat.

We see immediately that the definition of a stressor depends on the processing system that assigns meaning to it. The shock of an earthquake is a direct threat to many organisms, though not to a bacterium. The loss of a job is more acutely stressful to a salaried employee whose family lives month to month than to an executive who receives a golden handshake.

Equally important is the personality and current psychological state of the individual on whom the stressor is acting. The executive whose financial security is assured when he is terminated may still experience severe stress if his self-esteem and sense of purpose were completely bound up with his position in the company, compared with a colleague who finds greater value in family, social interests or spiritual pursuits. The loss of employment will be perceived as a major threat by the one, while the other may see it as an opportunity. There is no uniform and universal relationship between a stressor and the stress response. Each stress event is singular and is experienced in the present, but it also has its resonance from the past. The intensity of the stress experience and its long-term consequences depend on many factors unique to each individual. What defines stress for each of us is a matter of personal disposition and, even more, of personal history.

Selye discovered that the biology of stress predominantly affected three types of tissues or organs in the body: in the hormonal system, visible changes occurred in the adrenal glands; in the immune system, stress affected the spleen, the thymus and the lymph glands; and the intestinal lining of the digestive system. Rats autopsied after stress had enlarged adrenals, shrunken lymph organs and ulcerated intestines.

All these effects are generated by central nervous system pathways and by hormones. There are many hormones in the body, soluble chemicals that affect the functioning of organs, tissues and cells. When a chemical is secreted into the circulation by one organ to influence the functioning of another, it is called an endocrine hormone. On the perception of a threat, the hypothalamus in the brain stem releases corticotropin-releasing hormone (CRH), which travels a short distance to the pituitary, a small endocrine gland embedded in the bones at the base of the skull. Stimulated by CRH, the pituitary releases adrenocorticotrophic hormone (ACTH).

ACTH is in turn carried by the blood to the adrenals, small organs hidden in the fatty tissue on top of the kidneys. Here ACTH acts on the adrenal cortex, a thin rind of tissue that itself functions as an endocrine gland. Stimulated by ACTH, this gland now secretes the corticoid hormones (*corticoid*, from "cortex"), the chief among them being cortisol. Cortisol acts on almost every tissue in the body one way or another— from the brain to the immune system, from the bones to the intestines. It is an important part of the infinitely intricate system of physiological checks and balances by which the body mounts a response to threat. The immediate effects of cortisol are to dampen the stress reaction, decreasing immune activity to keep it within safe bounds.

The functional nexus formed by hypothalamus, pituitary and adrenal glands is referred to as the *HPA axis*. The HPA axis is the hub of the body's stress mechanism. It is implicated in many of the chronic conditions we will explore in later chapters. Because the hypothalamus is in two-way communication with the brain centres that process emotions, it is through the HPA axis that emotions exert their most direct effects on the immune system and on other organs.

Selye's triad of adrenal enlargement, lymphoid tissue shrinkage and intestinal ulcerations are due, then, to the enhancing effect of ACTH on the adrenal, the inhibiting effect of cortisol on the immune system and the ulcerating effect of cortisol on the intestines. Many people who are prescribed cortisol-type drugs in treatment for, say, asthma, colitis, arthritis or cancer are at risk for intestinal bleeding and may need to take other medications to protect the gut lining. This cortisol effect also helps to explain why chronic stress leaves us more susceptible to developing intestinal ulcers. Cortisol also has powerful bone-thinning actions. Depressed people secrete high levels of cortisol, which is why stressed and depressed postmenopausal women are more likely to develop osteoporosis and hip fractures.

This cursory description of the stress reaction is necessarily incomplete, for stress affects and involves virtually every tissue in the body. As Selye noted, "A general outline of the stress response will not only have to include brain and nerves, pituitary, adrenal, kidney, blood vessels, connective tissue, thyroid, liver, and white blood cells, but will also have to indicate the manifold interrelations between them."[4] Stress acts on many cells and tissues in the immune system that were largely unknown when Selye was conducting his pioneering research. Also involved in the immediate alarm response to threat are the heart, lungs, skeletal muscles and the emotional centres in the brain.

We need to mount a stress response in order to preserve internal stability. The stress response is non-specific. It may be triggered in reaction to any attack—physical, biological, chemical or psychological—or in response to any *perception* of attack or threat, conscious or unconscious. The essence of threat is a destabilization of the body's homeostasis, the relatively narrow range of physiological conditions within which the organism can survive and function. To facilitate fight or escape, blood needs to be diverted from the internal organs to the muscles, and the heart needs to pump faster. The brain needs to focus on the threat, forgetting about hunger or sexual drive. Stored energy supplies need to be mobilized, in the form of sugar molecules. The immune cells must be activated. Adrenaline, cortisol and the other stress substances fulfill those tasks.

All these functions must be kept within safe limits: too much sugar in the blood will cause coma; an overactive immune system will soon produce chemicals that are toxic. Thus, the stress response may be understood not only as the body's reaction to threat but also as its attempt to maintain homeostasis in the face of threat. At a conference on stress at the National Institutes of Health (U.S.), researchers used the concept of the stable internal milieu to define stress itself "as a *state of disharmony or threatened homeostasis.*"[5] According to such a definition, a stressor "is *a threat, real or perceived, that tends to disturb homeostasis.*"[6]

What do all stressors have in common? Ultimately they all represent the absence of something that the organism perceives as necessary for survival—or its threatened loss. The threatened loss of food supply is a major stressor. So is—for human beings—the threatened loss of love. "It may be said without hesitation," Hans Selye wrote, "that for man the most important stressors are emotional."[7]

The research literature has identified three factors that universally lead to stress: *uncertainty, the lack of information and the loss of control.*[8] All three are present in the lives of individuals with chronic illness. Many people may have the illusion that they are in control, only to find later that forces unknown to them were driving their decisions and behaviours for many, many years. I have found that in my life. For some people, it is disease that finally shatters the illusion of control.

Gabrielle is fifty-eight, active in a local scleroderma society. Her naturally large eyes are magnified by the effect of her skin being stretched tightly on her face, her smile a barely perceptible movement of her lips over perfect white teeth. Her narrow fingers shine with the waxy translucency characteristic of scleroderma, but they also display some of the deformity of rheumatoid arthritis. Several digits have "drifted" off centre and are swollen at the joints. Gabrielle was diagnosed with scleroderma in 1985. Usually the disease's onset is slow and insidious, but the first symptoms she experienced came on with flu-like suddenness—probably because in her case the scleroderma is associated with a more generalized rheumatic arthritis. "I was very, very ill for close to a year," she recalls.

"The first five or six months I was hardly able to get out of bed. It was an effort to get up and do anything because of pain everywhere there is a joint. I would respond to an anti-inflammatory or Tylenol 3 for maybe three or four weeks. Then it wouldn't be effective any more, so we would change and try something else. I was unable to eat. In five weeks I lost thirty pounds. I was down to ninety-one pounds. . . . I had read in different articles that people who come down with scleroderma are those who've always had to feel in control. All my life I'd been the one in charge, taking care of everything. Suddenly now with the disease you are totally out of control."

It may seem paradoxical to claim that stress, a physiological mechanism vital to life, is a cause of illness. To resolve this apparent contradiction, we must differentiate between *acute stress* and *chronic stress.* Acute stress is the immediate, short-term body response to threat. Chronic stress is activation of the stress mechanisms over long periods of time when a person is exposed to stressors that cannot be escaped either because she does not recognize them or because she has no control over them.

Discharges of nervous system, hormonal output and immune changes constitute the flight-or-fight reactions that help us survive immediate danger. These biological responses are adaptive in the emergencies for which nature designed them. But the same stress responses, triggered chronically and without resolution, produce harm and even permanent damage. Chronically high cortisol levels destroy tissue. Chronically elevated adrenalin levels raise the blood pressure and damage the heart.

There is extensive documentation of the inhibiting effect of chronic stress on the immune system. In one study, the activity of immune cells called natural killer (NK) cells were compared in two groups: spousal caregivers of people with Alzheimer's disease, and age- and health-matched controls. NK cells are front-line troops in the fight against infections and against cancer, having the capacity to attack invading micro-organisms and to destroy cells with malignant mutations. The NK cell functioning of the caregivers was significantly suppressed, even in those whose spouses had died as long as three years previously. The caregivers who reported lower levels of social support also showed the greatest depression in immune activity—just as the loneliest medical students had the most impaired immune systems under the stress of examinations.

Another study of caregivers assessed the efficacy of immunization against influenza. In this study 80 per cent among the non-stressed control group developed immunity against the virus, but only 20 per cent of the Alzheimer caregivers were able to do so. The stress of unremitting caregiving inhibited the immune system and left people susceptible to influenza.[9] Research has also shown stress-related delays in tissue repair. The wounds of Alzheimer caregivers took an average of nine days longer to heal than those of controls.

Higher levels of stress cause higher cortisol output via the HPA axis, and cortisol inhibits the activity of the inflammatory cells involved in wound healing. Dental students had a wound deliberately inflicted on their hard palates while they were facing immunology exams and again during vacation. In all of them the wound healed more quickly in the summer. Under stress, their white blood cells produced less of a substance essential to healing.

The oft-observed relationship between stress, impaired immunity and illness has given rise to the concept of "diseases of adaptation," a phrase of Hans Selye's. The flight-or-fight response, it is argued, was indispensable in an era when early human beings had to confront a natural world of predators and other dangers. In civilized society, however, the flight-fight reaction is triggered in situations where it is neither necessary nor helpful, since we no longer face the same mortal threats to existence. The body's physiological stress mechanisms are often triggered inappropriately, leading to disease.

There is another way to look at it. The flight-or-fight alarm reaction exists today for the same purpose evolution originally assigned to it: to enable us to survive. What has happened is that we have lost touch with the gut feelings designed to be our warning system. The body mounts a stress response, but the mind is unaware of the threat. We keep ourselves in physiologically stressful situations, with only a dim awareness of distress or no awareness at all. As Selye pointed out, the salient stressors in the lives of most human beings today—at least in the industrialized world—are emotional. Just like laboratory animals unable to escape, people find themselves trapped in lifestyles and emotional patterns inimical to their health. The higher the level of economic development, it seems, the more anaesthetized we have become to our emotional realities. We no longer sense what is happening in our bodies and cannot therefore act in self-preserving ways. The physiology of stress eats away at our bodies not because it has outlived its usefulness but because we may no longer have the competence to recognize its signals.

Like stress, emotion is a concept we often invoke without a precise sense of its meaning. And, like stress, emotions have several components. The psychologist Ross Buck distinguishes between three levels of emotional responses, which he calls Emotion I, Emotion II and Emotion III, classified according to the degree we are conscious of them.

Emotion III is the subjective experience, from within oneself. It is how we feel. In the experience of Emotion III there is conscious awareness of an emotional state, such as anger or joy or fear, and its accompanying bodily sensations.

Emotion II comprises our emotional displays as seen by others, with or without our awareness. It is signalled through body language— "non-verbal signals, mannerisms, tones of voices, gestures, facial expressions, brief touches, and even the timing of events and pauses between words. [They] may have physiologic consequences—often outside the awareness of the participants."[10] It is quite common for a person to be oblivious to the emotions he is communicating, even though they are clearly read by those around him. Our expressions of Emotion II are what most affect other people, regardless of our intentions.

A child's displays of Emotion II are also what parents are least able to tolerate if the feelings being manifested trigger too much anxiety in them. As Dr. Buck points out, a child whose parents punish or inhibit this acting-out of emotion will be conditioned to respond to similar emotions in the future by repression. The self-shutdown serves to prevent shame and rejection. Under such conditions, Buck writes, "emotional competence will be compromised. . . . The individual will not in the future know how to effectively handle the feelings and desires involved. The result would be a kind of helplessness."[11]

The stress literature amply documents that helplessness, real or perceived, is a potent trigger for biological stress responses. Learned helplessness is a psychological state in which subjects do not extricate themselves from stressful situations even when they have the physical opportunity to do so. People often find themselves in situations of learned helplessness—for example, someone who feels stuck in a dysfunctional or even abusive relationship, in a stressful job or in a lifestyle that robs him or her of true freedom.

Emotion I comprises the physiological changes triggered by emotional stimuli, such as the nervous system discharges, hormonal output and immune changes that make up the flight-or-fight reaction in response to threat. These responses are not under conscious control, and they cannot be directly observed from the outside. They just happen. They may occur in the absence of subjective awareness or of emotional expression. Adaptive in the acute threat situation, these same stress responses are harmful when they are triggered chronically without the individual's being able to act in any way to defeat the perceived threat or to avoid it.

Self-regulation, writes Ross Buck, "involves in part the attainment of *emotional competence,* which is defined as the ability to deal in an appropriate and satisfactory way with one's own feelings and desires."[12] Emotional competence presupposes capacities often lacking in our society, where "cool"—the absence of emotion—is the prevailing ethic, where "don't be so emotional" and "don't be so sensitive" are what children often hear, and where rationality is generally considered to be the preferred antithesis of emotionality. The idealized cultural symbol of rationality is Mr. Spock, the emotionally crippled Vulcan character on *Star Trek.*

Emotional competence requires

- the capacity to feel our emotions, so that we are aware when we are experiencing stress;
- the ability to express our emotions effectively and thereby to assert our needs and to maintain the integrity of our emotional boundaries;
- the facility to distinguish between psychological reactions that are pertinent to the present situation and those that represent residue from the past. What we want and demand from the world needs to conform to our present needs, not to unconscious, unsatisfied needs from childhood. If distinctions between past and present blur, we will perceive loss or the threat of loss where none exists; and
- the awareness of those genuine needs that do require satisfaction, rather than their repression for the sake of gaining the acceptance or approval of others.

Stress occurs in the absence of these criteria, and it leads to the disruption of homeostasis. Chronic disruption results in ill health. In each of the individual histories of illness in this book, one or more aspect of emotional competence was significantly compromised, usually in ways entirely unknown to the person involved.

Emotional competence is what we need to develop if we are to protect ourselves from the hidden stresses that create a risk to health, and it is what we need to regain if we are to heal. We need to foster emotional competence in our children, as the best preventive medicine.

4

Buried Alive

LEXA AND HER HUSBAND, PETER, wanted a second opinion. A death sentence had been pronounced on her, and they hoped I would be able to repeal it. Alexa was an elementary teacher in her early forties. In the year preceding our meeting, the small muscles in her hands had begun to shrivel up and she had increasing difficulty grasping objects. She also suffered inexplicable falls. She sought advice from Dr. Gordon Neufeld, a noted developmental psychologist in British Columbia whom she had come to know through his consulting work in the school system. Believing it was "only stress," she avoided considering a medical explanation.

Alexa forced herself to carry on with her professional duties; she struggled to maintain her routine beyond any reasonable point, well past the line most people would draw in taking care of themselves. "She worked incredibly long hours and was overextended," Dr. Neufeld recalls. "I've never seen anybody push herself to the extent that she did." Because she could barely hold pen or pencil, Alexa often stayed up long after midnight to complete her daily marking of student assignments. In the morning she would arise at five-thirty, in order to arrive at school early enough to scrawl the day's lesson on the blackboard, the chalk gripped in her closed fist. As her condition deteriorated further, she finally accepted a referral to an international authority on amyotrophic lateral sclerosis, Dr. Andrew Eisen. Electrophysiological testing and clinical examination left no doubt in Dr. Eisen's mind that the patient had ALS. At this point Peter and Alexa asked me to review the medical evidence, hoping I would discover something to challenge the specialist's opinion—or, more precisely, hoping I would support their belief that

the symptoms were purely stress related. The diagnosis was irrefutable—
as Dr. Eisen said, "a classic case."

In ALS the motor neurons, nerve cells that initiate and control muscle
movement, gradually die. Without electical discharges from the nerves,
the muscles wither. As the Web site of the ALS Society explains: "*A-myo-
trophic* comes from the Greek language. 'A' means no or negative. 'Myo'
refers to muscle, and 'trophic' means nourishment—'No muscle nourishment.' When a muscle has no nourishment, it 'atrophies' or wastes
away. 'Lateral' identifies the areas in a person's spinal cord where por-
tions of the nerve cells that nourish the muscles are located. As this area
degenerates it leads to scarring or hardening ('sclerosis') in the region."
        Initial symptoms depend on the area of the spinal cord or the brain
stem where the disease first strikes: people may experience muscle
twitching or cramps, loss of normal speech or difficulties swallowing.
Mobility and limb movement are eventually lost, as is speech, swallowing and the capacity to move air in and out of the lungs. Despite a few
reported cases of recovery, early death is usually inevitable. About 50 per
cent of patients succumb within five years, although some may survive
much longer. The British cosmologist Stephen Hawking, author of *A
Brief History of Time,* has lived with the diagnosis for decades—for reasons
that may emerge when we come to study his example. In contrast with
other degenerative diseases of the nervous system, ALS patients lose
muscle control without suffering intellectual decline. As a research paper
by Suzannah Horgan, a Calgary psychologist, puts it, "Most stories from
patients convey the strains of having to manage the combination of an
intact mind and an impaired body."[1]
        What causes the neurological degeneration from ALS is not known.
There is some evidence there may be immune system involvement,
including a dysfunction of the cells in the nervous system that have an
immune role. A class of cells called *microglia* serve a protective role in the
brain, but when hyperstimulated they may become destructive. An article
in *Scientific American* in 1995 cited tantalizing preliminary data pointing
to microglia as possible participants in multiple sclerosis, Parkinson's
disease and ALS.[2]
        Alexa and Peter were striking in their desperation to think their
way past their tragic situation. Peter, a retired engineer, would get

bogged down in arcane details of muscle electrophysiology, quoting research of dubious significance and proposing theories that would have made an expert's hair stand on end. He would often interrupt his wife when I asked her a question; she, in turn, would cast sidelong glances at him, as if for approval, as she gave her answers. It was evident that he found the prospect of Alexa's death unbearably frightening, and also that she appeared to deny the diagnosis more for his sake than her own. I felt as though I was engaged in conversation not with two separate individuals, but with one possessed of two bodies. "Alexa could not afford to think a separate thought," says Dr. Neufeld. "She could not afford to say anything about Peter that would have indicated she was a separate person from him."

Also painfully obvious was Alexa's inability to speak emotional language. She simply had no vocabulary to express her feelings directly: any question related to emotion would be answered by thoughts, delivered in a hyperarticulate but confused fashion. She seemed to perceive the world through abstract ideas instead of felt experience. "All of the emotions seemed completely frozen," confirms Neufeld.

What froze Alexa was her overwhelming fear of abandonment. Given up by her birth parents, she had never established a connection with her adoptive mother. "There was nothing in that relationship; it never worked," says Dr. Neufeld, who came to know Alexa closely in her last three years of life. "The adoptive mother had another child whom she favoured, and there was nothing Alexa could do, try as she might. She became estranged as an adolescent, finally, because she gave up. Until then, she worked desperately to make a connection with her adoptive mother and couldn't. It was a total vacuum. Alexa felt like there was a huge cavern where the sense of self should be." Her first marriage quickly fell apart. She grew up believing she had to take care of everybody. "There was never any respite in her," says Neufeld. "There was no internal resting place."

In a 1970 research article, two psychiatrists at the Yale University School of Medicine, Walter Brown and Peter Mueller, recorded dramatically similar impressions of ALS patients. "They invariably evoked admiration and respect from all staff who came into contact with them," wrote Drs. Brown and Mueller. *"Characteristic was their attempt to avoid asking for help."*[3] This Yale study of ten patients employed interviews, clinical evaluations and self-administered psychological tests. The authors concluded that people with ALS seemed to have two life-long patterns distinguishing them: rigidly competent behaviour—that is, the inability to ask for or receive help, and the chronic exclusion of so-called negative feelings. "Hard, steady work without recourse to help from others was pervasive," the study notes. There seemed to have been a "habitual denial, suppression or isolation of . . . fear, anxiety, and sadness. . . . Most expressed the necessity to be cheerful. . . . [Some] spoke casually of their deterioration or did so with engaging smiles." The conclusions of this 1970 Yale paper were not confirmed by a study seven years later, at the Presbyterian Hospital in San Francisco. One might say the jury is out, except that the Yale study is consistent with everything that can possibly be read about ALS patients, observed about them, or told by clinicians working with them. Studies in psychology—an art trying desperately to dress itself up as a pure science—often find only what the particular researchers have the eyes to see.

"Why Are Patients with ALS So Nice?" was the title of an intriguing paper presented by neurologists from the Cleveland Clinic at an international symposium in Munich a few years ago.[4] It discussed the impression of many clinicians that people with Lou Gehrig's disease nearly all seem to "cluster at the MOST PLEASANT end" of the personality spectrum, in contrast to persons with other diseases.

At the Cleveland Clinic, a major referral centre for amyotrophic lateral sclerosis, the protocol for suspected ALS patients begins with electrodiagnostic testing (EDX). By measuring electrical conductivity, EDX detects the viability or death of motor neurons, the nerve cells that act on muscle fibres. Niceness is commonly perceived by staff to be a feature of the ALS personality, reports Dr. Asa J. Wilbourn, senior author of the paper. His article noted: "This occurs so consistently that whenever the EDX technologists have completed their work and deliver the results . . . they usually accompany it with some comment [e.g., 'This patient cannot have ALS, he (or she) is not nice enough. . . . '] In spite of the briefness of their contact with the patients, and the obvious unscientific method by which they form their opinions, *almost invariably these prove to be correct.*"

"The interesting thing in Munich was that when we presented our paper, everybody came around," says Dr. Wilbourn. " 'Oh yeah,' people commented, 'I've noticed that—I've just never thought about it.' It's almost universal. It becomes common knowledge in the laboratory where you evaluate a lot of patients of ALS—and we do an enormous number of cases. I think that anyone who deals with ALS knows that this is a definite phenomenon."

Similar patterns emerge from my personal encounters with ALS patients in private practice and in palliative care. Emotional repression—in most cases expressed as niceness—can also be found on exploring the lives of famous persons with ALS, from the physicist Stephen Hawking, the baseball great Gehrig, to Morrie Schwartz, the professor whose television appearances on Ted Koppel's show made him a much-admired figure in the last months of his life and whose story and wisdom form the subject of the best-seller *Tuesdays with Morrie*. In Canada, Sue Rodriguez, a person with ALS, gained national prominence with her determined legal battle for her right to assisted suicide. In the end not even a Supreme Court decision could deny her that right. Her story is congruent with what the lives of these others also teach us.

The life histories of people with ALS invariably tell of emotional deprivation or loss in childhood. Characterizing the personalities of ALS patients are relentless self-drive, reluctance to acknowledge the need for help and the denial of pain whether physical or emotional. All these behaviours and psychological coping mechanisms far predate the onset of illness. The conspicuous niceness of most, but not all, persons with ALS is an expression of a self-imposed image that needs to conform to the individual's (and the world's) expectations. Unlike someone whose human characteristics emerge spontaneously, the individual seems trapped in a role, even when the role causes further harm. It is adopted where a strong sense of self should be—a strong sense of self that could not develop under early childhood conditions of emotional barrenness. In people with a weak sense of self, there is often an unhealthy fusion with others.

The example of New York Yankees first baseman Lou Gehrig is instructive. Gehrig earned the sobriquet "the iron horse" for his implacable refusal to remove himself from the lineup regardless of illness or injury. In the 1930s, long before the days of sophisticated physiotherapy and sports medicine, he set a record for consecutive games played—2,130—that would stand for the next six decades. He seemed to feel that his prodigious talents and dedicated play when healthy were not enough, and he was too dutiful toward his fans and employers to ever take time off. Gehrig was caught up, according to his biographer, "in his self-designated role as a loyal son, loyal team player, loyal citizen, loyal employee."[5]

A teammate recalled Gehrig's participation in a game despite a broken middle finger on his right hand. "Every time he batted a ball it hurt him. And he almost got sick to his stomach when he caught the ball. You could see him wince. But he always stayed in the game." When his hands were X-rayed, it was found that every one of his fingers had been broken at one time or another—some more than once. Long before ALS forced him to retire, Gehrig had sustained seventeen separate fractures in his hands. "He stayed in games grinning crazily like a macabre dancer in a gruelling marathon," someone wrote. The contrast between Gehrig's unsparing attitude toward himself and his solicitude toward others was glaringly evident when a Yankee rookie was weak from a heavy cold. Placating the annoyed team manager, Gehrig took the young man home to be cared for by his mother, who treated the "patient" to hot wine and put him to bed in her son's room. Lou slept on the couch.

Gehrig has been described as a quintessential "mama's boy." He lived with his mother until his marriage, in his early thirties—a union the mother accepted only with marked ill grace.

Stephen Hawking was diagnosed at the age of twenty-one. His biographers write: "During his first two years at Cambridge, the effects of the ALS disease rapidly worsened. He was beginning to experience enormous difficulty in walking, and was compelled to use a stick in order to move just a few feet. His friends helped him as best they could, but most of the time he shunned any assistance. Using walls and objects as well as sticks, he would manage, painfully slowly, to traverse rooms and open areas. There were many occasions when these supports were not enough. . . . On some days Hawking would turn up at the office with a bandage around his head, having fallen heavily and received a nasty bump."[6]

Dennis Kaye, a Canadian who died of ALS, published *Laugh, I Thought I'd Die* in 1993. His book has the reader doubled over with laughter, even knowing the author's fate—exactly as Kaye had intended. Like several other writers with ALS, he remained undaunted by the exorbitant physical demands of writing without the use of his fingers or hands.

"Let me start by saying that ALS is not for the faint of heart," he begins his chapter titled "Lifestyles of the Sick and Feeble." "In fact, I only recommend it to those who truly enjoy a challenge." Kaye tapped out his volume with a stick fastened to his forehead. Here is his description of the "ALS personality": "One seldom sees words like 'deadbeat' or 'lazy' used in the same sentence as ALS. In fact, one of the only traits ALSers seem to share is an energetic past. In almost every case, victims were either classic over-achievers or chronic workaholics. . . . I've been called a workaholic, and I suppose if the work-boot fits . . . but technically, even though I worked all the time, I was never driven by an addiction to work so much as an aversion to, perhaps even a disdain for, boredom."[7]

Another Canadian with ALS, Evelyn Bell, authored her book *Cries of the Silent* by wearing a laser light attached to a special glass frame, shining it on a spelling board, painstakingly pointing out each letter of each word to volunteer assistants for transcription. For her, too, such zealous dedication to a goal was not new. She relates that she had lived her life "at a feverish pace." She was the mother of three children while building a successful business career: "It was a challenge to juggle homemaking, parenting, business, gardening, interior decorating and chauffeuring, but *I loved the roles and performed them with great intensity. . . . *During the years of raising a family, my Nutri-Medics business grew extensively and I enjoyed many company cars and numerous trips to foreign lands. I reached many levels of success in the business, being top achiever in Canada for a number of years. I felt I wanted to be a success at parenting and everything I did." With unconscious irony, Evelyn Bell reports all this just after writing that "*we knew we could always replace money but not our health or our marriage.*"[8]

Disease frequently causes people to see themselves in a different light, to reassess how they have lived their lives. A sudden realization hit Dennis Kaye one day as—with "glib satisfaction"—he watched his father, and two employees, doing work that he, Dennis, had always unquestioningly performed on his own. "Before long," he writes, "satisfaction turned to frustration. . . . Almost all my accomplishments were in one way or another connected not to *my* aspirations, but to the aspirations of my father. I don't want this to turn into an Oprah-style confession, but from the time I was a kid working my summer holidays, I'd been helping my father meet his goals and obligations. Except for a couple of years in my late teens, I'd spent the past fourteen years meeting someone else's deadlines. . . . Suddenly, in the blink of an eye, I found myself pushing thirty and facing a deadline of my own . . . the ultimate deadline."

The same compulsive sense of duty to others is evident in Laura, an ALS patient I met recently. A sixty-five-year-old former teacher of dance, Laura greets me at the door of her magazine-classic wood and glass West Coast home. Even leaning on her walker for support, she displays the grace and elegance of the ballet dancer. She was diagnosed with ALS four years ago, while undergoing chemotherapy for breast cancer. "I went to a concert," she relates, "and I couldn't clap all of a sudden. My fingers were cramping and they just weren't as dexterous as they usually are. It seemed to get worse as I went through the chemo. I had several bad falls; one time I broke my cheekbone and my eye socket." Laura's speech is halting, but the cadences of lively humour and a love for life can still be heard in the near-monotonous flow of her delivery.

Laura's medical troubles came on after a tense year during which she worked hard at the new bed-and-breakfast business she established in the home she shares with Brent, her second husband. "I had always wanted to open a B and B," she says. "I found this place, but there was stress because we had to come up with more money than we could really afford. I felt guilty that Brent had to subsidize my financial venture. That first year was difficult, decorating the rooms. We built the carriage house. I ran the business, made the house, as well as decorating. It was practically a year to the day we moved in that I discovered the lump." The ALS diagnosis followed a few months later.

Laura exemplifies just how impossible people with ALS find it to let go of self-imposed responsibilities long after their bodies have signalled rebellion. When we conducted our interview, the housekeeper for the bed and breakfast was away in Europe. "It turned out that 70 per cent of our clientele are repeats," says Laura. "You get to know them as friends, you know. I've been feeling guilty because we said we are not going to take any guests for the month while Heidi was gone. But last weekend we had three rooms occupied because I couldn't say no. They are repeats and I enjoy seeing them. And next week we have one repeat coming who's been here a dozen times, a corporate guest."

"How about saying," I suggest, "'Dear corporate guest: I have this condition that makes life very difficult for me. I am not up to the work involved in looking after people.'"

"I could say that. But the gal is coming, and I really enjoy her. She knows my condition, and she says, 'I'll clean up my own room, and I'll get a bowl of cereal in the morning.' That's what they all say, but I can't let them do that. Because I've never served a bowl of cereal for breakfast."

"You still wouldn't be serving one. They'd be serving it themselves."

Hearty laughter. "You make it sound so simple. I'd have to take a course, or maybe get some counselling with you."

Laura's guilt around saying no to other people's perceived needs was inculcated at an early age. Her mother developed breast cancer when Laura was twelve and died four years later.* From adolescence Laura was responsible for the care of her sister and brother, respectively five and ten years younger than she is. Even before then she was habituated to anticipating her parents' wishes.

"My mother was a dance teacher, so I danced as a very young child and all through my life. I went into the Royal Winnipeg Ballet, but I ended up being too tall, so I opened a dance school with a friend and taught children."

"It's a very demanding life, ballet. Did you enjoy it as a child?"

"Sometimes. Sometimes I resented it. I resented not being able to go with my friends to a show on a Saturday afternoon, or it always seemed I was missing birthday parties."

"How did you deal with that?"

"My mother would give me a choice, and *I think I would go dancing because I knew she preferred that I do that.*"

"What about what you preferred?"

"I would have liked to go with my friends."

After her mother's death, Laura functioned as the woman of the house, not only as caregiver to her siblings but, in some ways, also as companion to her father. "He'd say, 'What are you doing tonight, Laura?' I'd say, 'I'm going to a show with Connie,' my best friend. He'd say, 'Oh, I think I'll get a babysitter and come with you.' All

---

* *A gene for breast cancer runs in Laura's family. Her sister was also diagnosed, six months before Laura. Breast cancer will be the subject of a later chapter.*

my friends came to our house 'cause they loved my dad. He was just great with everyone."

"How did you feel about your dad hanging out with you and your girlfriends?"

"Well, what kind of teenager wants their dad hanging around!"

"Did you ever say, 'Dad, I just want to be with my friends'?"

"No . . . I didn't like it, but I didn't want to hurt his feelings."

Laura's first husband, whom she married to escape the family home, was a compulsive womanizer. He left her when she was pregnant with their third child, on her own, without any financial support. They had been childhood sweethearts.

"He was having affairs? For how long did you endure it?" I wonder.

"Four years. I had two children, and I believed in marriage." Laura slowly lifts a napkin to her eyes to wipe away some tears. "I've never talked about this."

"It's still very painful for you."

"I don't know why, it was a hundred years ago. . . . Sorry, I do get emotional."

"What's that like for you to get emotional?"

"Annoying, because it doesn't do any good."

"Is being emotional something you've found uncomfortable in your life?"

"Well, if you're emotional, it's usually because something bad or sad has happened, so why would you like being emotional?"

In a sense, Laura is right. For the child it is no relief to feel sadness or anger if no one is there to receive those emotions and to provide some comfort and containment. Everything had to be held in rigidly. The physical rigidity of ALS may well be a consequence. There is perhaps only so much energy the nervous system can expend pushing down powerful emotions that cry out for expression. At some point in particularly susceptible individuals, it seems reasonable to suppose, nerves may lose the ability to renew themselves. Could ALS be a result of an exhausted nervous system no longer being capable of replenishing itself?

"Why has the fact that ALS patients, as a group, are strikingly congenial not been discussed in the literature?" asked the Cleveland neurologists in their Munich presentation. "Probably the principal reason is that it is based on subjective assessments, which lack a means of scientific verification. Thus, according to our psychiatric colleagues, 'niceness' is extremely difficult to quantify." Perhaps if researchers took greater care to obtain patients' life histories, much useful information now being missed would be forthcoming. The examples in this chapter illustrate that.

Rage and anguish exist underneath the veneer of niceness, no matter how sincerely a person mistakes the facade for her true self. "My mother is still alive, and I love her dearly," says the sister of a man diagnosed with ALS two years ago, "but she is very domineering, superficial in her understanding of emotions and insensitive to other people's needs and wants. She does not allow you to have your own self. It was very difficult to find your own identity with my mother. When I consider my brother's illness, I think we all did our work to figure out how to become separate individuals. It's been hard, but we did—except my brother, who somehow didn't. He said to me last time I was there—I'm fifty-four now, and he's forty-six—'I hate Mom.' And yet, he is the one who is the nicest to my mother of us all. He will go there—he has ALS and can hardly walk—but he will take soup to her. When he is in my mom's presence he will be a cute little boy—the good little kid he always was, and I was not."

Joanne, a beautiful thirty-eight-year-old with black hair and luminous, sad blue eyes, was admitted to our palliative unit for terminal care a few months before her death. She had been a dancer. The sudden and bewildering refusal of her limbs to obey her will on the dance floor was traced to the onset of amyotrophic lateral sclerosis. Proud of her innate ability to move freely and creatively, Joanne experienced this diagnosis as the most devastating blow imaginable. "I'd rather die of some horrible cancer," she said. Already at the end stages of the disease, she wanted me to promise to kill her when the time came. I guaranteed we would not let her suffer pain or breathlessness. That was a promise I could in good conscience make without compromising the principled rejection of euthanasia shared by most doctors and nurses who do palliative work.

You can come to know people quickly and deeply when you look after them during their time of dying. Joanne and I had many talks. "All my life," she once told me, "ever since childhood, I have been having this dream of being buried alive. I lie in my underground coffin, closed in, unable to breathe. When I was diagnosed three years ago I went to the office of the ALS Society for information. There on the wall was a poster that read 'Having ALS Is Like Being Buried Alive.'"

I do not believe Joanne's recurrent nightmare was either coincidence or preternatural premonition. The image of being alone, confined, desperate and doomed, unheard by anyone, was the psychological truth of her childhood existence. She never experienced herself as an alive and free being in her relationships with her parents or siblings. I could only speculate what stresses over how many generations had finally created that situation for her in her family of origin. As it was, neither her parents nor her brothers and sisters visited during her terminal phase. A new family of devoted caregivers accompanied Joanne during her final weeks on earth and were with her to her dying breath. She was deeply asleep during her final days. The promise was kept: she did not suffer at the last.

Sue Rodriguez, the Victoria woman whose court-defying suicide was carried out in the presence of a member of Canada's Parliament, was also emotionally isolated from her family. Her biographer, the journalist Lisa Hobbs-Birnie, describes the day Rodriguez's diagnosis with ALS was confirmed:

> Sue felt her knees buckle, her legs turn to water. She knew what ALS was, had seen the documentary on the physicist-astronomer Stephen Hawking, knew his condition, tried to imagine her own life inside a body that couldn't sit up, walk, talk, laugh, write or hug her child. . . . She leaned against a wall. She became aware of a terrible sound, as primal as the cry of a wounded animal, unlike anything she'd heard before. She realized only slowly, from the horrified expressions of passersby, that it was coming from her own mouth. . . .
>
> She phoned to tell her mother and step-father, Doe and Ken Thatcher. Doe said: "Ken and I thought it might be that." Sue felt abandoned, and gave way to uncontrollable grief.[9]

Sue was the second of the five children born to her parents within ten years. She was always the outsider. Her mother somehow believed that Sue made this choice: "It almost seemed," she said, "from the moment she was born she didn't feel part of the family in the same way as the others did. The illness only made it worse." Mother and daughter had only occasional telephone contact during the final months of Sue's life. Doe was characterized by her daughter and others as "not the caregiving type."

"The mother's brusque reaction when Sue called from the hospital with her diagnosis," writes Hobbs-Birnie, "was typical not only of Doe's lack of caregiving skill, but of the kind of interaction mother and daughter had. Things did not improve as Sue's disease progressed." Emotional communication was foreign to the Rodriguez family, according to her brother, fourteen months her junior. He was the only sibling to maintain any regular contact with his dying sister. Most of the family, he said, preferred not to show their feelings.

This is not some bizarre, unfeeling group of human beings here. The problem was not a lack of feeling but an *excess* of painful, unmetabolized emotion. The Rodriguez family dealt with emotional hurt by repressing it. Generations of family history had brought them to that coping pattern. Sue's father, Tom, dead of alcohol-induced cirrhosis of the liver at age forty-five, had been an earlier victim of this surfeit of pain. He was a man of low self-esteem, all his life dominated by others.

What drove a terminally ill Sue Rodriguez, the mother of a young child, to expend her diminishing physical and psychic resources on highly public court battles and media campaigns that taxed her vital energies to the limit? An articulate woman with an engaging personality and a beautiful smile, she became a hero to many who saw her as a crusader of indomitable courage and spirit. She was popularly viewed as someone fighting for her right to die at a time and in the manner of her own choosing.

There was always more to the Sue Rodriquez story than the simple issue of autonomy in death, though this was the part of her drama that caught the imagination of the public. Behind the popular facade of a confident and determined fighter, Ms. Rodriguez was a frightened and lonely person with a very fragile support system, alienated from her estranged husband and from her family. It was a multi-layered scenario. As usual, the most public layer was also the most superficial one.

The biographer believes Sue Rodriguez was "a woman of strong convictions and a powerful sense of self. She had control over her life and preferred to have control over her death." As with all ALS patients, the reality was rather more contradictory. Strong convictions do not necessarily signal a powerful sense of self: very often quite the opposite. Intensely held beliefs may be no more than a person's unconscious effort to build a sense of self to fill what, underneath, is experienced as a vacuum.

Her history of deeply troubled personal relationships indicates that Sue Rodriguez had never been in control of her life. She had filled roles without ever being close to her real self. Her anguished question to the court and the public—"Who owns my life?"—was a summation of her whole existence. Her fight for control in death turned out to be her final and greatest role. By the time her legal case opened, writes Lisa Hobbs–Birnie, "Sue Rodriguez was fast becoming a national figure. *She slid into the role as if her entire life had been a preparation for it, which indeed it had.*"

When Sue Rodriguez was diagnosed with ALS, in her first despair she compared the impossibility of her situation with what she perceived were the relative advantages of fellow ALS sufferer Stephen Hawking. Writes Hobbs–Birnie, "She was given pamphlets on palliative care, and these pamphlets described patients who were 'surrounded by loving family' or who found joy in 'living a life of the mind.' What loving family? she thought. What life of the mind? Let a genius like Stephen Hawking live a life of the mind. But me, if I cannot move my own body, I have no life."

If Stephen Hawking's public status as a latter-day Einstein may be questioned by science cognoscenti, no one disputes his brilliance, originality of thought or intellectual fearlessness. There is universal admiration for the indomitable will that has sustained his life and work since a slight speech impediment signalled the onset of amyotrophic lateral sclerosis when he was only twenty years old. Diagnosed in 1963, Hawking was given the medical prognosis that he had, at most, two years to live. He has been near death on at least one occasion, ill with pneumonia and in a coma on a trip to Switzerland. Yet four decades after his diagnosis, paralyzed, wheelchair bound and completely dependent physically, he has, nonetheless, just published his second best-selling book. He has travelled ceaselessly around the world, a lecturer in great demand despite his inability to utter a word in his own voice. He has been the recipient of many scientific honours.

Although there are exceptions, the course of ALS is generally predictable. The vast majority of patients die within ten years of diagnosis, many much sooner. Very rarely people do make recovery from what seems like ALS, but it is extremely unusual for a person to live with its ravages for as long as Stephen Hawking has, continuing not only to work but to function at a high level. What has enabled him to confound medical opinion and those grim statistics?

We cannot understand Hawking's course as an isolated clinical phenomenon, separated from the circumstances of his life and relationships. His longevity is, without doubt, a tribute to his spirited determination not to allow the disease to defeat him. But I also believe that Sue Rodriguez's bitter comparison was correct: the young Stephen had access to invisible resources denied to most people with ALS. Given the nature of ALS as a disease that destroys body while leaving the intellect intact, an abstract thinker was in an ideal position to "live a life of the mind." Unlike the athletic rock climber and former marathoner Rodriguez and unlike the dancers Laura and Joanne, Hawking did not see his body's deterioration as impairing the role that he chose for himself. On the contrary, it may have enhanced it. Prior to his diagnosis and its attendant debility, he had been somewhat aimless, his shining intellectual gifts notwithstanding.

Hawking had always possessed tremendous cognitive and mathematical capacities and confidence, but he never seemed to feel comfortable in his body. "He was eccentric and awkward, skinny and puny," write Michael White and John Gribbin in *Stephen Hawking, A Life in Science.* "His school uniform always looked a mess and, according to his friends, he jabbered rather than talked clearly. . . . He was just that sort of kid—a figure of classroom fun, teased and occasionally bullied, secretly respected by some and avoided by most." He did not look to fulfill the expectations those who had glimpsed his true abilities held for him. The young Stephen, it appears, was the chosen bearer of the frustrated ambitions of his father who was evidently determined that his son would succeed at educational and social goals he, the father, had never quite attained. One goal was to have Stephen attend one of England's most prestigious private schools. The ten-year-old-boy was entered for the Westminster School scholarship examination: "*The day of the examination arrived, and Stephen fell ill.* He never sat the entrance paper and consequently never obtained a place at one of England's best schools."

One may assume, of course, that this untimely illness was purely coincidental. We may also see it as the child's only way of saying no to parental pressure. Given the Hawking family's penchant for privacy, the facts would be difficult to discern. What we do know is that later on, with the young Hawking no longer living at home and at liberty to follow his preferences, these appeared to be more of a social than academic nature. Stephen engaged in a fair bit of indolence and alcohol consumption, with avoidance of classes or studying—those classic forms of passive resistance in college. For a while his academic career looked in jeopardy, and briefly he considered entering the civil service. It was only after his diagnosis that he began to focus his phenomenal intelligence on his work: elucidating the nature of the cosmos, bridging the theoretical gaps between Einsteinian relativity theory and quantum mechanics. With his physical disability, he was freed from many of the tasks of teaching and administration other scientists have to shoulder. His biographers write: "Some have attributed his great successes in cosmology to this enhanced cerebral freedom, yet others have claimed that the turning-point in the application of his abilities was the onset of his condition, and that before then he was no more than an averagely bright student."

That latter point is difficult to accept, but even Hawking has acknowledged that it was only after the onset of his illness that he began to exert himself at anything: "I . . . started working for the first time in my life. To my surprise, I found I liked it. Maybe it's not really fair to call it work. Someone once said, scientists and prostitutes get paid for doing what they enjoy."

Not much insight there about prostitutes, but it is clear Hawking has been in the extremely fortunate position of being able to pursue a genuine vocation, despite his extreme physical limitations.

The other indispensable factor Hawking possessed and Rodriquez missed was the unconditional emotional support and practical caring of a loved one. For Stephen the source of this nurturing was his wife, now his former wife, Jane Hawking. In essence, she decided to devote her life to him—at great personal cost to herself, as she would come to learn. The two met just before Stephen's diagnosis with ALS and were married shortly afterwards. Due to her own history, Jane was primed to accept the role of devoted and selfless caregiver. I write *selfless* here advisedly: there was lacking in her a developed, autonomous sense of self, and thus she completely identified with her role as Stephen's nurse, mother and guardian angel. "I wanted to find some purpose to my existence," she recalls in her 1993 memoir, *Music to Move the Stars*, "and I supposed I found it in the idea of looking after him." When she doubted her ability to fulfill that daunting task, friends told her, "If he needs you, you must do it." She took it on.

The two young people did not just join each other as equals in a spousal partnership: they fused. They became one body, heart and soul. Without the subordination of Jane's life and independent strivings to his, Stephen likely would not have survived, let alone succeeded to such a spectacular degree. His biographers assert that "without the help that Jane gave him, he almost certainly would not have been able to carry on, or had the will to do so."[10]

The relationship worked as long as Jane accepted her self-abnegating position and the one-way flow of psychic energy between them, from wife to husband. The couple loved each other, but she would come to feel used. She recounts a strange incident when, in 1965, she arrived at her fiancé's apartment with a broken arm in a cast: "He was actually expecting that I would put my secretarial skills to good use by typing out a job application for him. The look of horrified dismay that spread across his face as I walked into his room with my left arm bulging beneath my coat in a white plaster cast dashed all my hopes of even the merest display of sympathy."

The episode encapsulated the nature of their relationship: she was the ever-available, unspeaking and compliant mother/nanny figure whose services are expected, taken for granted and noticed only in their absence. She travelled the world with her husband, daily confronting and overcoming myriad difficulties that were only much later—and even then only partially—eased once he became an internationally famous and high-earning author. She felt herself gradually disappear as an individual. She was sucked dry, sensing herself becoming a "brittle, empty shell, alone and vulnerable," and nearly suicidal. Hawking, for his part, reacted to her strivings for independence with disdain and finally with the rage of a child deserted by his mother. The wife was eventually supplanted by a nurse who left her own husband to marry the scientist. Jane, too, had found another love. It was only this outside relationship that, in the final years of the marriage, allowed her to continue to serve Stephen as long as she did.

Hawking's vocation and the unstinting support of his wife were accompanied by something else that has probably aided his survival: the liberation of his aggression by his illness. The "niceness" of most ALS patients represents more than the innate goodness and sweetness of some human beings; it is an emotion *in extremis*. It is magnified out of healthy proportion by a powerful suppression of assertiveness.

Assertiveness in defence of our boundaries can and should appear aggressive, if need be. Hawking's intellectual self-assuredness became the ground for that aggression to manifest itself, particularly after the onset of his physical decline. Jane Hawking notes in her memoir that "curiously, as his gait became more unsteady so his opinions became more forceful and defiant."

Like that of all the ALS sufferers we have met, Hawking's personality has been characterized by intense psychological repression. In his family of origin, healthy vulnerability and emotional interaction appear to have been perceived as foreign. At the supper table, the Hawkings would eat without communicating, each head lowered into reading matter. Stephen's childhood home was in a state of physical neglect that went beyond eccentricity to indicate an emotional distance on the part of both parents. His biographers relate, "Neither Isobel nor Frank Hawking semed to care too much about the state of the house. Carpets and furniture remained in use until they began to fall apart; wallpaper was allowed to dangle where it had peeled through old age; and there were many places along the hallway and behind doors where plaster had fallen away, leaving gaping holes in the wall."

Of Stephen's father, White and Gribbin write that he was a remote figure, "significant in Stephen's childhood and adolescence by his absence." According to Jane, the Hawkings regarded "any expression of emotion or appreciation as a sign of weakness, as loss of control or a denial of their own importance. . . . Strangely, they seemed ashamed of demonstrating any warmth."

After Stephen and Jane married, his family withdrew from active involvement with his care, a fact Jane could barely fathom, let alone accept. Besides her responsibilities toward her husband, she also had full care of their three children. His refusal to acknowledge the pressures placed on her by his illness—and her compliant subjection to that attitude—meant that she never received any respite. "I was at the breaking-point," she recalls, "but still Stephen was determined to reject any proposals which might have suggested that he was making concessions to the illness. These were the proposals which might have relieved the children and me of some of the strain." He simply refused to discuss any problem, relying on Jane's willingness to absorb all the resultant stress. "He had never liked to admit to emotions," writes Jane, "regarding them as the fatal, irrational flaw in my character." Her attempts to gain support from her husband's family were met with cold incomprehension, even hostility. "You see," her mother-in-law once told her, "we have never really liked you, Jane; you do not fit into our family." This after decades of self-effacing service to her son.

Has it been shown in this chapter that ALS is caused by, or is at least potentiated by, emotional repression? That it is rooted in childhood emotional isolation and loss? That generally—even if not always—it strikes people who lead driven lives and whom others consider to be very "nice"? Until our understanding of the mind/body complex is more advanced, this must remain an intriguing hypothesis but a hypothesis one would be challenged to find any exceptions to. It seems far-fetched to suppose that such frequently observed associations can be all a matter of pure coincidence.

A mind-body perspective may help those afflicted with ALS who are willing to look at some very painful realities fully and unflinchingly. In rare instances, people do seem to get over symptoms diagnosed as ALS. It would be worthwhile investigating such cases to find out why. One example is reported by Dr. Christiane Northrup in *Women's Bodies, Women's Wisdom*:

> Dana Johnson, a researcher friend of mine and a registered nurse, even recovered from Lou Gehrig's disease by learning to respect all aspects of her body.
>
> After she had had the disease for some years, she began to lose control over her breathing muscles as well as the rest of her body. Her breathing difficulties made her think she was going to die. But she decided at that point that she wanted to experience unconditional

love for herself at least once before dying. Describing herself as a "bowl of Jell-O in a wheelchair," she sat every day for fifteen minutes in front of a mirror and chose different parts of herself to love. She started with her hands, because at that time they were the only parts of herself that she could appreciate unconditionally. Each day she went on to other body parts. . . .

She also wrote in a journal about insights she had during this process, and she came to see that since childhood she had believed that in order to be of service, acceptable to others, and worthy of herself, she had to sacrifice her own needs. It took a life-threatening disease for her to learn that service through self-sacrifice is a dead end.[11]

According to Dr. Northrup, her friend healed through the conscious daily practice of emotional self-inventory and of self-love that, little by little, "unfroze" each part of her body. Had I read such a story when I graduated from medical school, I would have dismissed it out of hand. Even now, the scientifically trained physician in me would like to see direct proof that ALS was legitimately diagnosed in this case. In palliative work I once saw a person admitted for "respite care" who had convinced herself and her circle of friends that she suffered from ALS, despite the electrodiagnostic testing and neurological findings having all been, repeatedly, perfectly normal. The friends scarcely believed me when I informed them that the invalid they had been assiduously caring for was, from the narrow physical point of view, as healthy as they were.

Today I do not find Dr. Northrup's report impossible to credit. It accords with my understanding of this disease. There was an intriguing incident in the story of Alexa, the teacher whose husband, Peter, could not accept the diagnosis of ALS. It revealed the potential of something that, perhaps, may have been. The psychologist Gordon Neufeld managed on only one occasion to see her alone, without her spouse. "It was absolutely clear to me that her emotions were tied up, that she had lost her vitality," Dr. Neufeld says. "There was a two-hour session when Peter was away, and she grieved intensely about her life and about her illness. It made a huge difference to her. The physiotherapist saw her right afterwards and was amazed that her muscle tone was so much better. But I could never meet with her alone again, and I could never get her to that place again. The window just shut."

5

Never Good Enough

FOR SEVEN YEARS, MICHELLE HAD a lump in her breast. Periodically, it grew or shrank, but it never caused her or her physicians any concern. "Then all of a sudden it got really hard, got hot and started to grow almost overnight," the thirty-nine-year-old Vancouverite says. A biopsy revealed that the tumour was malignant, and Michelle believes she knows why: stress. "It wasn't until I shocked the hell out of my life that it changed," she says. "I quit my job, without any income to go to. . . . My emotional state was horrible at the time. A lot of things hit me all at once, not only financial." Michelle had a lumpectomy and was relieved to learn that her lymph glands were free of cancer. The surgery was followed by chemotherapy and radiation, but no physician ever asked her about what psychic stresses she might have suffered before the onset of her malignancy or what unresolved issues she had in her life.

Breast cancer patients often report that their doctors do not express an active interest in them as individuals or in the social and emotional context in which they live. The assumption is that these factors have no significant role in either the origins or the treatment of disease. That attitude is reinforced by narrowly conceived psychological research.

An article in the *British Medical Journal* reported on a five-year study of more than two hundred women with breast cancer that aimed to determine whether a recurrence of cancer can be triggered by severe life events, such as divorce or the death of someone close. The authors concluded that "women with breast cancer need not fear that stressful experiences will precipitate a return of their disease."[1] Dr. Donna Stewart, a professor at the University of Toronto and chairwoman of women's issues for the University Health Network, commented that the study's results "made sense."

Dr. Stewart was the lead author of a study published in 2001 in the journal *Psycho-Oncology*. Nearly four hundred women with a history of breast cancer were asked what they thought had caused their malignancy. Forty-two per cent cited stress—much more than other factors such as diet, environment, genetics and lifestyle.[2] "I think it reflects what's going on in society in general," Dr. Stewart says. "People think stress causes everything. The evidence for stress is pretty low. And the evidence for hormones and genetics is pretty high."

Yet Michelle and the many other women who suspect a strong relationship between stress and their breast cancer have science and clinical insight on their side. No other cancer has been as minutely studied for the potential biological connections between psychological influences and the onset of the disease. A rich body of evidence, drawn from animal studies and human experience, supports the impression of cancer patients that emotional stress is a major contributing cause of breast malignancy.

Contrary to the assertions of the Toronto researchers, the "evidence for genetics" is not high. Only a small minority of women are at high genetic risk for breast cancer and only a small minority of women with breast cancer—about 7 per cent—acquire the disease for genetic reasons. Even for those genetically predisposed, environmental factors must be involved, since far from everyone with one of the three genes known to be associated with breast cancer will actually develop a malignant tumour. In the vast majority of women or men diagnosed with breast cancer, heredity makes little or no contribution.

It is artificial to impose a separation between hormones and emotions. While it is perfectly true that hormones are active promoters or inhibitors of malignancy, it is not true that their actions have nothing to do with stress. In fact, one of the chief ways that emotions act biologically in cancer causation is through the effect of hormones. Some hormones—estrogen, for example—encourage tumour growth. Others enhance cancer development by reducing the immune system's capacity to destroy malignant cells.

Hormone production is intimately affected by psychological stress. Women have always known that emotional stress affects their ovarian function and their menstrual cycles—excessive stress may even inhibit menstruation.

The body's hormonal system is inextricably linked with the brain centres where emotions are experienced and interpreted. In turn, the hormonal apparatus and the emotional centres are interconnected with the immune system and the nervous system. These are not four separate systems, but one super-system that functions as a unit to protect the body from external invasion and from disturbances to the internal phys-iological condition. It is impossible for any stressful stimulus, chronic or acute, to act on only one part of the super-system. What happens to one will affect all. In chapter 7 we will examine the workings of this super-system more closely.

Emotions also directly modulate the immune system. Studies at the U.S. National Cancer Institute found that natural killer (NK) cells, an im-portant class of immune cells we have already met, are more active in breast cancer patients who are able to express anger, to adopt a fighting stance and who have more social support. NK cells mount an attack on malignant cells and are able to destroy them. These women had significantly less spread of their breast cancer, compared with those who exhibited a less assertive attitude or who had fewer nurturing social connections. The researchers found that emotional factors and social involvement were more important to survival than the degree of disease itself.[3]

Many studies, such as the one reported in *The British Medical Journal* article, fail to appreciate that stress is not only a question of external stimulus but also of individual response. It occurs in the real lives of real persons whose inborn temperament, life history, emotional patterns, physical and mental resources, and social and economic supports vary greatly. As pointed out in chapter 3, there is no universal stressor.

In most cases of breast cancer, the stresses are hidden and chronic. They stem from childhood experiences, early emotional programming and unconscious psychological coping styles. They accumulate over a lifetime to make someone susceptible to disease.

Michelle grew up in a home where both parents were alcoholics. She now believes that her malignancy is related to early experiences that shaped how she has faced life. She has tried to cope in ways that, unconsciously, increased the stress load she had to carry for many years—for example, by taking care of other people's emotional needs rather than her own. "I've been confused all my life," she says, "and I think my cancer had to do with confusion. . . . As much as I believe and understand my parents loved us the best way they knew how, it was the most confusing relationship and family environment because they were alcoholics, and still are. They're unloving even though there is love."

Research has suggested for decades that women are more prone to develop breast cancer if their childhoods were characterized by emotional disconnection from their parents or other disturbances in their upbringing; if they tend to repress emotions, particularly anger; if they lack nurturing social relationships in adulthood; and if they are the altruistic, compulsively caregiving types. In one study, psychologists interviewed patients admitted to hospital for breast biopsy, without knowing the pathology results. Researchers were able to predict the presence of cancer in up to 94 per cent of cases judging by such psychological factors alone.[4] In a similar German study, forty women with breast cancer were matched with forty controls similar in age, general health history and lifestyle considerations. Again, on psychological grounds the researchers were 96 per cent successful in identifying who was and who was not diagnosed with breast cancer.[5]

As a man, Melvin Crew* was at first embarrassed to learn of his diagnosis with breast cancer but decided that "there's no sense just lying back and letting the disease consume you." Now, several years after mastectomy, chemotherapy and radiation, he jokes about it. "At least if you fall down, you can't go tits up because I only have one, you know."

Fifty-one-year-old Crew was diagnosed in 1994 immediately after a highly stressful period in his life, including a brush with the law over a fishing infraction, public embarrassment, humiliation at work and undue pressure from his employer. He had been on a boat with ten other men and had caught three fish. When fisheries officers made a raid at his house, he gave them a statement.

---

* Mr. Crew has already gone public with news of his breast cancer. Unlike the women interviewed, he does not need his identity protected.

"Two other chaps and myself took the brunt; the rest of the fellows denied it. It was hard on my family to have my name plastered across the papers—coast-guard employees charged with illegal fishing—and the whole works. And then, when I did go back on one of the other coast-guard ships, there was the heckling from the other crew members and the jokes that were made. . . . All the fellows at work said I should have denied it."

This pressure was all the more stressful for Melvin, who describes himself as having always prided himself on his conscientiousness. "Some of my co-workers have said to me, you know, you take your job too serious. They think that I don't relax enough."

"Do you ever feel you're doing the work that other people should have done?" I ask.

"Yes, you do more than your share. That's probably just my nature—you know, you don't want to be looked upon as a slackass."

"If other people don't do their share, one solution is to do it for them. The other is to get angry about it."

"If you get angry, it's like adding fuel to the fire. You have your conscientious workers, and you have your workers that just go with the flow. I did feel angry sometimes. Well, if you express it, you just bring on more problems with the workforce."

The source of his hyper-conscientiousness became evident when I asked Melvin about his childhood.

"Was there much affection in your home?"

"Yes. My father was proud of my sister and me and our accomplishments in life. She's a teacher. My father was an engineer, and I, of course, followed in his footsteps. Got my engineer's licence, and my father was really proud of my being an aircraft engineer."

"Warmth and affection have nothing to do with achievement: they are there regardless of achievement, just because the parents are emotionally connected with the child. But your answer had to do with accomplishment. I wonder why that is?"

"Well, my father was always proud of us."

"What about your mom—what kind of affection did you get from your mom?"

"Not overly affectionate. We loved our parents, and I feel they certainly provided a good upbringing for us. A good home."

About 1 per cent of breast cancer patients are males. Their emotional histories parallel those of the women with the same disease. David Yeandle, a Toronto policeman, has had four separate cancers: in one of his kidneys, his breast and twice in his bladder. His upbringing was also characterized by a lack of warmth. Born in 1936, David was three when the Second World War broke out. His sister was born in 1940.

"My father was a warehouseman, and my mother worked at Cadbury's chocolates. . . . I grew up during the war and actually didn't see a lot of my parents. My mother was out during the day, and my sister and I used to take care of ourselves until she came home.

"You must mean that as a very small child, you used to take care of your sister."

"Yes."

David recalls his parents' marriage as an unhappy one. "They weren't a loving couple," he says. "My dad did his thing, and my mother did hers. My dad, most evenings, would go out and shoot pool with his friends. I didn't have a lot of respect for my mother. She always expected me to give more than I could. I guess I wasn't a brilliant student. And my mother always saw herself much better than what she was. She was working class, the whole family was, but she always gave the impression to people that we were better than what we were. You had to perform to her standards."

"When you were upset as a child, when you felt not understood, when you felt emotionally troubled, whom did you talk to about it?"

"Actually, you kept it within yourself. Dad was never there to talk to, and I certainly wouldn't discuss it with my mother, because her favourite expression was 'Oh, you're being silly.' I never showed anger with my parents. It was something you just didn't do. I hold a lot of anger inside me."

"Extreme suppression of anger" was the most commonly identified characteristic of breast cancer patients in a 1974 British study. The investigators looked at a consecutive series of 160 women admitted to hospital for breast biopsy. All subjects were given a detailed psychological interview and self-administered questionnaire. For corroboration, spouses or other family members were also interviewed, separately. Since the psychological testing took place before the biopsy, neither the women nor the interviewers could have prior knowledge of the ultimate diagnosis. "Our principal finding was a significant association between the diagnosis of breast cancer and a behaviour pattern, persisting throughout adult life, of abnormal release of emotions. This abnormality was, in most cases, extreme suppression of anger and, in patients over 40, extreme suppression of other feelings."[6]

A 1952 psychoanalytic evaluation of women with breast cancer had come to similar conclusions. These patients were said to demonstrate "an inability to discharge or deal appropriately with anger, agressiveness, or hostility (which, in turn, was masked by a facade of pleasantness)." The researchers felt that patients' unresolved conflicts were "manifested through denial and unrealistic self-sacrificing behaviours."[7]

The research conducted by Dr. Sandra Levy and her associates at the U.S. National Cancer Institute on the relationship between natural killer cell activity and emotional coping patterns in breast cancer concluded that *"suppression of anger and a passive, stoic response style seem to be associated with biological risk sequelae."*[8]

Repression of anger increases the risk for cancer for the very practical reason that it magnifies exposure to physiological stress. If people are not able to recognize intrusion, or are unable to assert themselves even when they do see a violation, they are likely to experience repeatedly the damage brought on by stress. Recall, from chapter 3, that stress is a physiological response to a perceived threat, physical or emotional, whether or not the individual is immediately aware of the perception.

"I obviously struggle with the first question that everyone I know who has had cancer asks: 'What did I do to deserve this? Why me?' Did I do something wrong? I went over and over everything. I'm not the one that was supposed to get breast cancer. I breast-fed my children to twenty-one months. I smoked a little, only when I was young. I didn't drink too much. I exercised. I watched the fat in my diet. This wasn't supposed to happen to me." The speaker is Anna, a mother of three who was in her mid-forties when the suspicious lump was found eight years ago. Anna has one of the breast cancer genes.

Even in the small minority of cases where it is a major predisposing factor, heredity cannot by itself explain who gets breast cancer and who does not. DNA testing has shown that Anna inherited the breast cancer gene from her father. Other relatives with the same gene, older than she is, have not developed breast cancer. Anna is convinced that stress was instrumental in the development of her cancer. Her first husband, a businessman, mistreated her emotionally throughout her marriage. By the time the relationship ended, she was also being physically abused. "If you ask me why I got cancer, I would tell you it's because I allowed myself to be so destroyed in that marriage. I was this close to suicide more times than I . . .

"I didn't have enough self-respect. Am I good enough yet, could you love me yet? I married my mom. He was exactly like my mother. I was never good enough. When I look back, I think, How could I have stayed in such a marriage? I've cried plenty over that at the therapist's. How could I have done that to my soul, because that's what I hurt. I hurt the essence of who I was. And I think I hurt my body too.

"Finally, I felt there was very little of me left in my world. I was taking eight prescription drugs a day for depression, anxiety, insomnia, aches and pains, bowel problems. It was either die, or get out. At that point, the self-preservation kicked in and I got out."

Anna fits that pattern of "unrealistic self-sacrificing behaviours" noted in the 1952 psychoanalytic study of breast cancer patients. She is the only one among four siblings to take responsibility for her father, now in his eighties.

"He pulls on my heartstrings. I feel awful when he has a problem. I feel terrible when he phones up and says, 'I'm so lonesome—I've got nowhere to go and nothing to do today.' My sister, who I think is a bitch, says, 'Hey, that's his problem, he had a million choices and chances.'

"We went through a hysterical scene with him a year and a half ago when I asked him to go into respite care for one month. He'd been in the hospital, and I had been at the hospital all day every day, sitting there for hours and hours and hours. He came out and I felt like I was having a nervous breakdown from looking after him. I pulled the cancer card—the big card—and said, 'Dad, look'—with the social workers and everyone—'I've had cancer and I have to look after myself. I cannot look after you like this. Please (I'm crying by this point because I am the crier in the family), please, stay here for one month.' He said, 'No. Why should I? I don't want to.'

"The social worker and the head of the program are saying to him, 'Mr. W., no one wants to come into a seniors' home. Could you do it for your daughter? Look at your daughter—she's crying and is really having a hard time. She needs time with her husband; she needs a break.' 'No, I won't,' he said. 'Why should I?'

"When I had my double mastectomy, I asked my brother and sisters if they would look after Dad for a while. 'I can't have him over for dinner for a couple of months,' I told them. 'I need to recover.' Within ten days he was here for dinner because no one else was looking after him. And nobody even notices."

"What you've assumed toward your dad is a maternal role. Which is also why you've been taken for granted. Mother is taken for granted. Mother is like the world—she's just supposed to be there and provide."

"Absolutely. My brother does the same thing—I'm my brother's mother as well. When he phones, my kids say, 'Uncle Don must have a problem because he's phoning again.' He suffers from depression; he goes through relationships like you wouldn't believe. He's here day and night when there's a problem. Then he won't return my phone calls for months. He can't be bothered.

"He came once the whole time I had chemotherapy. I sat down with him about a year and a half after my diagnosis and my chemo was over. That was my first experience with trying to say what I needed really clearly. I said, 'Don, I need something from you. When I go to the cancer clinic for checkups, I need you to ask me how it came out. It's really important to me. I need you to ask me what happened when I went.' He leaned back and said, 'I need something from you too,' and launched into this long thing about his relationship with this girl that was breaking up. I just sat there and thought that he just didn't get it at all. You're right—at some point I realized, I'm mom."

Anna felt repeatedly abandoned by her mother, who favoured her older sister. "I didn't have a mom. My mom checked out," she says, "and basically didn't like me, so I really couldn't afford to lose my dad, too. Kids are smart enough to understand they need a parent. And my father loved me the wrong way." From adolescence on, Anna noticed her father casting undisguised sexual glances at her, particularly at her breasts.

"I picked up something from him, which I spent most of my life denying until I got into some counselling. He didn't, as far as I know, do anything, but he wanted to. He looked . . . There was a sexual intensity that for an eleven- or twelve-year-old girl . . . I'm hypersensitive to anything coming from men. Anything. But for a young woman to let herself believe that her father feels like that is really hard. I mean, Christ almighty, you make a million excuses for why it's not real. My sister, though—there's no way she would ever show up in a T-shirt when Dad was around.

"My father is probably the only person who doesn't know I've had my breasts removed because I've never told him. I don't think anyone else is going to. He knows I had an operation that was cancer related. He asked Steve (Anna's second husband), 'Is this something to do with the breast?' and Steve said, 'Yes, it's a continuation of the previous thing.' Dad has never said anything to me. Through my chemo he was so ignorant and shitty to me. He'd come in the front door and say, 'Go put your wig on. You don't look pretty.' I'd say, 'You know what, I'm really, really sick and I just rolled out of bed to answer this door.' Only I wouldn't say it calmly like that—I'd get hysterical.

"I was driving him home recently, and he said, 'I've got to speak to you about something. I know you're not the person I should tell, but I have no one else.' Then he launches into this thing—he's eighty-two years old—about how his girlfriend doesn't want to have sex with him. 'Men have needs.' That's something he taught me early. A wife must—he told me straight up—never say no to her husband when he wants sex because if she does, he has the right to get it somewhere else. It's your duty to provide sex. Here he is telling me that he wants to have sex and his girlfriend won't and he has needs and what is he supposed to do. I'm sitting there thinking, This is so inappropriate—you should not be talking to your daughter about this."

"Mind you . . . you could also say, 'Dad, I don't want to hear this.'"

"But then he'd be embarrassed. He'd feel ashamed and think he'd done something. It's my job to not let him feel ashamed.

"At what point do I get to say, 'I don't want to.' These are strange words for me, in any situation. I'll lie to people, I won't answer the phone, I'll say 'I'm moving to Tibet so I can't take part in that'—I'll do anything but say 'I don't want to.' And when there's no lie that comes to mind, I just take it all on."

The straightforward connection between childhood experience and adult stress has been missed by so many researchers over so many years that one almost begins to wonder if the oversight is deliberate. Adults with a history of troubled childhoods may not encounter more serious losses than others do, but their ability to cope will have been impaired by their upbringing. Stress does not occur in a vacuum. The same external event will have greatly varied physiological impact, depending on who is experiencing it. The death of a family member will be processed in a markedly different way by someone who is emotionally well integrated and in a supportive relationship than it will be by a person who is alone or—like Anna prior to her therapy—tormented by chronic guilt due to childhood conditioning.

One person whose true childhood history would likely be missed on self-administered questionnaires of breast cancer patients is former U.S. first lady Betty Ford. Mrs. Ford has written courageously in her autobiography, *The Times of My Life*, about her alcoholism and her efforts at healing after a family intervention by her husband, her children and others. She has been equally forthright in revealing her diagnosis and treatment for breast cancer, but—it appears from her published accounts—when it comes to her childhood she is still wearing rose-coloured glasses. She is typical of the person who represses her own feelings in order to preserve a sense of idyllic relationship with the parent.

Betty Ford, married to a decent but ambitious politician whose career dominated her life, was emotionally deprived in her spousal relationship. "I probably encouraged my husband to drink. He was such a reserved man it was difficult for him even to tell me he loved me—he had proposed by saying, 'I'd like to marry you.'" For many years she suffered from what were clearly stress-related low-back pains, diagnosed as "osteoarthritis" and treated with painkillers and tranquilizers. She also drank heavily to soothe physical and emotional pain. Ford describes herself as filled with self-doubt and unable to assert herself:

> I was convinced that the more important Jerry became, the less important I became. And the more I allowed myself to become a doormat—I knew I was a doormat to the kids—the more self-pity overwhelmed me. Hadn't I once been somebody in this world?
>
> Underneath, I guess I didn't really believe I had been somebody. My career with Martha Graham hadn't been a huge success—I had talent as a dancer, but I wasn't a great dancer—and my confidence had always been shaky.

I couldn't accept that people liked me for myself. And I was self-conscious that I didn't have a college degree. . . .

Uneducated. No Pavlova. And not half the woman my mother had been. I was measuring myself against impossible ideals—Martha or my mother—and coming up short. That's a good recipe for alcoholism.

My mother was a wonderful woman, strong and kind and principled, and she never let me down. She was also a perfectionist, and tried to program us children for perfection. My mother never came to us with her problems, she just shouldered them. And she was my strongest role model, so when I couldn't shoulder my problems, I lost respect for myself. No matter how hard I tried, I couldn't measure up to my own expectations.[9]

The former first lady seems blind to her own disclosures here—about the way she experienced her childhood, about how her relationship with her mother and, no doubt, with her father, of whom she says very little—shaped her personality and coping style. She does not see that surrendering herself to her husband's needs and expectations—becoming a "doormat"—resulted from childhood conditioning. The emotional repression, the harsh self-judgment and the perfectionism Betty Ford acquired as a child, through no fault of her own, are more than a "good recipe for alcoholism." They are also a "good recipe" for cancer of the breast.

6

You Are Part of

This Too, Mom

N *LOCK ME UP OR LET ME GO,* her second book of memoirs, Betty Krawczyk writes about the death from breast cancer of her twenty-seven-year-old daughter, Barbara Ellen:

The last migraine I had was in the palliative care unit, almost three years ago, when the doctor in charge told me that I should tell Barbara Ellen it was okay for her to die.

"She wants your permission to die," he said gently. We were in a private room reserved especially for people like me. The most wretched people of the earth.

"To hell with that!" I flung at him, shocked and horrified at the very suggestion. "She doesn't have my permission to die! I forbid it. . . ."

I had broken down at that point and was sobbing wildly. The doctor waited patiently. He was used to this reaction. That was his job.

"Mrs. Krawczyk, I think you understand that Barbara Ellen's suffering will simply increase now, by the hour."

"She is not suffering! She has the butterfly in her arm. She talked to her sisters and her father this morning, she saw friends just yesterday, she was talking to her little boy, and hugging him. . . ."

"That was a gift. A gift she gave loved ones. To tell everybody good-bye. You're the only one she hasn't told good-bye. She wants to do this now. She wants your permission to leave. . . ."

"Oh, please, don't! Who do you think you are, God? How do you know this is the hour of her death?"

And then I was reduced to begging. "Give me a few more days, please. Please put the IV back in. . . ."

"She doesn't want it. You have to be strong enough to give your daughter what she needs right now. She needs you to help her, to let her go; that's the only way you can help her now, to let her go."

The headache was so bad I thought I might expire before Barbara Ellen did. But I didn't. . . . By the following evening I . . . had recuperated enough to tell my daughter that if she was tired of being sick and wanted to go, I would no longer try to keep her. She held my hand and told me she would wait for me wherever it was that she was going, and she died that morning, in my arms, her sister Marian holding her, too, her father also by her side.[1]

I was the palliative physician in that scene. I well recall Barbara Ellen, huddled in her hospital bed under the window, in the first room on the right of the hall as you entered the ward from the elevator. Slight to begin with, she had been reduced to waif-like size by her terminal cancer. She said very little, and she seemed sad. I had no knowledge of her history, except for the essential details of her disease. She had been diagnosed with inflammatory breast cancer, a type that strikes young women and has a dismally poor prognosis. She had elected to refuse all conventional medical treatment—not an entirely unreasonable decision, considering her diagnosis, but highly unusual. Such decisions always involve more than the bare medical facts, and my sense was that this young woman felt quite isolated—had felt that way all her life. At times I just wanted to cradle and comfort her in my arms, as one would an infant or small child.

I had talked with Barbara Ellen after morning rounds on the day Betty depicts in her memoir. "How much longer do I have?" she asked.

"Not long. How does it feel to you?"

"I've had enough. Are you giving me anything to keep me alive?"

"Only the IV. Without the fluids you would die in a day or two. Would you like us to stop it?"

"My mother couldn't handle that."

"I get the feeling you always took care of her in some ways, so it may be difficult for you to do what you want now. But you don't need to take care of her any more. What would you do if you just took care of yourself?"

"I would take out the IV."

"I respect your mother's feelings. This is extremely hard on a parent—I can only imagine how unbearably difficult. But you are my patient here, and my primary responsibility is to you. If you wish, I will speak with her."

Recently Betty Krawczyk and I met again to talk about her daughter's life and death. We had conversed briefly after Barbara Ellen died, when Betty was grieving and attempting to comprehend why her daughter had died so much before her time. I had recounted for her my understanding about the possible connection between a stressful early childhood and an increased risk for the later development of cancer. Soon afterwards, I received in the mail a copy of her first volume of memoirs: *Clayoquot: The Sound of My Heart*. Inside the cover was this inscription: "Herewith my book. It explains something of my relationship with my daughter who died of breast cancer April 30 in your unit." Having read that book, I hoped Betty would agree to be interviewed for *When the Body Says No*. As it turned out, Betty had been thinking of me, having just written the passage quoted above. She was interested in learning more about my perspective and hoped I might help her understand better some of the things Barbara Ellen had said in the last six months of her life.

It was no ordinary discussion Betty and I had, but Betty is no ordinary woman. She is well known in British Columbia and beyond for her activism in environmental causes. The title of her first book refers to an internationally renowned rain-forest preserve on the West Coast, Clayoquot Sound, threatened some years ago by logging interests. In September 2001 seventy-three-year-old Betty was incarcerated four and a half months for criminal contempt of court, following another logging protest.

Although *Clayoquot* is mostly about Betty's experiences as an environmental crusader, she also gives a vivid and honest history of her personal life. With four husbands and eight children, she's had an eventful life. Now Betty acts as surrogate mother to Barbara Ellen's son, Julian, who was only two when his mother passed away.

Barbara Ellen gave vent to frequent expressions of deep anger at her mother in the final six months before she died. It is that anger Betty was still struggling to understand.

Betty Krawczyk was born in southern Lousiana, which, at that time, she says, was "mostly one big swamp." "I wasn't raised to be a protestor," she writes in *Clayoquot*. "I was raised a poor, country, southern white woman."

> Memory is so selective, so subjective. At a sibling confab several years ago we were tickled and somewhat amazed to learn that we each, my brother and sister and I, had felt the others to be favored in the family. I know I felt the other two to have been favored. Actually, I still do. My brother was the older, and the only boy, so he got most of the attention. What was left went to my sister because she was the baby and delicate to boot. I was a big, healthy girl who could amuse herself, so nobody took any special notice of me. Which was just fine as far as I was concerned.
>
> You really didn't want my father to notice you. If he did, you were in trouble. Not that he beat any of us ever, but the threat was always there. We were there to be seen not heard, and seen as little as possible. My mother was different. She was warm and loving. Although I always knew she favored my brother and sister, she was so full of love some of it slopped over on me, too. After I grew up I once confronted my mother with my secret knowledge, and she was hurt and astonished and insisted that if she paid more attention to the other two, it was because they needed her more than I did, that I was always more emotionally independent.[2]

Despite this apparent emotional independence, the young Betty suffered "wild nightmares and nervous imaginings in the dark." She left home early, marrying "the first grown man who came to court who could actually prove he was financially solvent." In short order, she left her husband, but not before bearing three children. "He was a bit of a compulsive collector of intact hymens. He couldn't seem to stop after we got married. He finally collected one too many."

Three more marriages and five more children followed in the next two decades. Barbara Ellen was the seventh among them, born just before Betty moved to Canada in 1966, "six kids in tow," and her third marriage on the verge of breaking up. They lived in Kirkland Lake, Ontario. Her husband, a college instructor, was an emotionally distant workaholic who also drank. "I didn't like John when he drank," she writes. "He had a tendency to get impossibly self-righteous and accusatory. So I found myself avoiding the same social situations I had originally reached out for. And my depression deepened. . . . I began to look at John and wonder who he actually was. . . . I thought that first winter in Kirkland Lake would never end and that spring would never come. Actually, spring never did come. . . . I think the two most frustrated people in that non-existent spring were me and the baby, Barbara Ellen."

Betty found a way out of her relationship with her husband by falling in love with his department head at the college and relocating with him to British Columbia. It was mostly here that Barbara Ellen grew up, although there were moves back and forth between Eastern and Western Canada, and between the United States and Canada.

Betty's fourth marriage also failed, but over the years she found a truer sense of herself as a person, as a woman and as an activist.

Barbara Ellen was a sensitive child with health problems. At the age of four, she began to have vomiting spells that nobody seemed able to diagnose. These bouts recurred intermittently over the years, and Betty feels now they were related to stresses in her daughter's life. As a young adult, Barbara became addicted to narcotic painkillers and tranquilizers that she would inject into her body. Right up to the time of her diagnosis with breast cancer, she was fighting her addiction to drugs. With no experience of stability, she was unable to establish an intimate, ongoing relationship with a man: she went from one relationship to another. Julian was born when Barbara Ellen was twenty-five, but when she married shortly afterwards, it was not to her child's father. "That marriage didn't last long," says Betty. "Martin was not able to cope with being married and having a little stepson."

Barbara was highly intelligent, sensitive and creative. A dancer, at one point she operated a ballet school for children. She was taking care of Julian and doing some teaching of dance classes in Vancouver when she discovered her cancer.

"She told me she had had this mammogram, and they just wanted to do a mastectomy. She wasn't willing to accept that. Barbara had a keen intellect. She researched all the material on the kind of cancer she had and investigated the treatment outcomes among her age group in the U.S. and Canada. She didn't like the way it looked. 'I am not going to go through all that,' she said. 'I don't want to be sick, I don't want to be mutilated, I don't want all this chemo stuff. I'm going to treat it holistically and do the best I can with it.' She asked that John and I support her decision and try not to interfere."

"How was that for you?"

"It was horrible. Immediately, I wanted to do something. I tried to pressure her to look at some other options, and then she was just very, very angry and adamant and yelled at me—she'd never yelled at me before. She was angry with me the whole last, I would say, six months of her life. Before, she wouldn't stay mad; when she was angry with me, she would just say, 'Okay, Mom, you want to think that, you think that,' and she'd slam her door or something, but that would be it."

"That's not exactly an expression of anger—mostly of defeat and frustration."

"She was always hurt by me for some reason, and I don't know why. I think I was a terrible parent for this child. My personality was hurtful to her."

"You're full of tears here. Are you still feeling guilt about it?"

"Maybe not so much guilt as a feeling that why couldn't they have given her to someone else who could have dealt with her. She was an extraordinary child in her sensitivity to the world, her understanding of the world, in her gentleness with the world."

"Gentleness . . . what was she like as a child?"

"She was very precocious. Wherever I took her, people were impressed with her demeanour and level of—I don't want to say that she acted adult—but at her level of comprehension of the adult world."

"How about emotionally?"

"Emotionally? She was a very loving and affectionate child. She was quite gentle and was always very loved by everyone, was always the teacher's pet. Other kids didn't seem to resent it, though."

"Do you have any sense at all that anybody ever tried to abuse her?"

"There was one incident. We had been to Louisiana visiting my mother and sister. My sister had these four boys. One boy was a year older than Barbara and bigger. Barbara would have been about twelve. She didn't tell me about this. It wasn't until we got back to California that she told Margaret, her sister. Margaret came and told me that this cousin tried to get on top of Barbara. They were the only two at home.

Barbara was very angry about it. I remember asking Margaret, 'Why didn't she come tell me?' and she said, 'She thought because Doris is your sister that it would cause a big ruckus between you two.'"

Betty and I then talked about Barbara's illness and death. At the time Barbara was diagnosed with cancer, Betty was running in a provincial election for the Green Party. She resigned her candidacy to spend time with her ailing daughter. I asked if she had found that difficult.

"It wasn't that hard. My feeling was that we needed each other. But there was something in my personality that Barbara always found irritating. My voice was too loud for her, my actions too flamboyant. I was too much for her more delicate constitution—that's the only way I can describe it. I'm too loud and too definite in my opinions and too aggressive in my actions. She had the opposite personality of liking to think about things and being quiet and trying to have a more holistic view of other people's personalities."

"It sounds like she thought you were more judgmental than she wanted you to be."

"She always accused me of being judgmental. I stayed awhile and she told me to go. She would always tell me when she was tired of me and she needed to rest because she found me tiring."

"This is in the last months?"

"Yes."

"Why do you think that is? You can't be tiring. There's no such thing as a tiring person."

"My personality would tire her after a while—it was too intense."

"When does one get tired?"

"When you've been working. So you think it was work for her to be with me."

"She had to work too hard around you."

"Aha . . ."

"Now you're wondering why I'm saying that. You'd be very unusual to be open to hearing this, but your whole life has been a search for truth. I know and understand that. Look, Barbara came along in your life when there was just no stability at all."

"That's right."

"You were going through the end stages of your relationship with John when you got pregnant with her, and you felt totally alone. You didn't feel partnered and you began to realize that while this guy was interesting intellectually, emotionally you were quite alone. Your way of leaving the relationship was to get involved with Wally. Then you make this flight to Western Canada with the kids in tow. What ends up happening is that John gets custody of everybody except Barbara Ellen. She had an awfully huge void to fill in your life all of a sudden, right from the beginning of her life.

"The nature of stress is not always the usual stuff that people think of. It's not the external stress of war or money loss or somebody dying, it is actually the internal stress of having to adjust oneself to somebody else. Cancer and ALS and MS and rheumatoid arthritis and all these other conditions, it seems to me, happen to people who have a poor sense of themselves as independent persons. On the emotional level, that is—they can be highly accomplished in the arts or intellectually—but on an emotional level they have a poorly differentiated sense of self. They live in reaction to others without ever really sensing who they themselves are.

"Barbara's going from one man to the other shows she hadn't enough of a sense of self to hold on to. As soon as one relationship is over, she had to get into another in order to feel okay about herself. The addictions enter into this as well.

"She comes along in your life when you are particularly emotionally needy and exhausted. I think her precocious intellectual development is what happens to bright and sensitive kids when the emotional environment isn't able to hold them enough; they develop this very powerful intellect that holds them instead. Hence their intellectual maturity and their ability to relate to adults. People would tell me as a child how mature I was. I always thought I was, because in that mode you can seem highly mature. But then when I look at myself emotionally, I've been very immature. I'm fifty-eight now and still trying to grow up."

"This is very interesting."

"What doesn't develop in one area will overdevelop in another, if the kid has the brains for it. Barbara develops a huge intellect in order to feel comfortable. I believe that's because you were not able to give her the emotional sustenance that she needed when she was small."

"I don't think so either."

"When the parent can't put in the work to maintain the relationship, then the child has to. She does so by being a good girl. She does it by being precocious, by being intellectually mature. When she reaches the age of abstract thought, around age thirteen or fourteen, when these connections in the brain actually happen, all of a sudden she becomes your intellectual sounding board. The relationship is based not on her needs but more on yours. With the incident of that boy trying to climb on her, she protects you from her emotional pain by not telling you. She doesn't let you know about it. She is taking care of you.

"She wants to keep peace in the family. That's not the child's role. The child's role is to go to her mother and say, 'This bastard tried to climb on top of me! To hell with whether there is peace or not!' I know that's what you would've wanted her to do. None of this is deliberate. It all goes back to your own experience as a child.

"I've had very similar interactions with my eldest son as you describe with Barbara. He said to me at one point, 'Dad, I don't know where you end and I begin.' That's just how it is. I've always said that I'm not worried my kids will be angry with me, I'm worried they won't be angry enough.

"What you were finally seeing in Barbara's last six months of life is that she was beginning to set boundaries. She was saying no, and the anger that she had repressed was coming out."

"Right . . ."

"This is how I perceive it. The people that I see with cancers and all these conditions have difficulty saying no and expressing anger. They tend to repress their anger or, at the very best, express it sarcastically, but never directly. It all comes from the early need to build the relationship with the parent, to work at the relationship.

"I think for Barbara it was a lot of work to maintain the relationship with you. I recall just very gingerly raising the issue. She indicated to me that there was something going on, but she also didn't want to talk very much. She was very much pulled into herself—I was a total stranger to her. She wasn't about to open up to me."

"It wasn't easy for her to open up. In the last months she would actually ask for me to come and smoke a joint with her, so then we could be relaxed and talk," Betty says.

"How was that?"

"It was good because she would talk about herself. She would say, 'I feel that I don't know what cancer is, but it's here and it seems like it's been visited on me.' She said, 'I've invited the cancer into my body.' I remember being horrified and saying, 'Barbara, I don't understand that.' She said, 'Well, it's because I experience it as part of my own life and that you're a part of this too, Mom. You have your own part of my cancer.'

"You know something else, Gabor—she saw somebody the night before she died. She said there was a man who'd come to take her, and she told him she wasn't ready. The next night, she said to me, 'That man—I want him to come.' I said, 'What man? Do you want me to call the doctor?' She said, 'No, the man who came for me and I told him I wasn't ready.' She said that she was ready now.

"I had told her a few hours before that if she was tired of being sick, she didn't have to hold on any longer. I'd said, 'Okay,' and it was then she told me this about the man. She told me that she was ready for him now, and she died at eight that morning. Have you ever read any Kubler-Ross stuff? You know where she says about escorts . . . people who come for us as we die. It was so weird. It really made the hair stand up on the back of my neck."

"Why is that weird for you?"

"Well, do you mean there really is an angel of death?"

"Does it have to be like that? The mind has an experience, and we translate it into an image. There is a deeper sense of something that's happening, but the mind can only experience it in terms of thoughts and images."

Betty had one final question. "Why can't parents see their children's pain?"

"I've had to ask myself the same thing. It's because we haven't seen our own. When I read your book, *Clayoquot*, I saw the evidence in your writing that you hadn't recognized your own pain yet. It would not be possible for you to clearly see Barbara's, either.

"If you think of it only in terms of you and Barbara, you're going to feel more guilt—you may accuse yourself of things that wouldn't be fair to you. The fact is, you are the product of a certain upbringing and a certain kind of life. Your life has always been about trying to find yourself and about trying to find truth in the world. It's been a real struggle.

It's amazing what you've done, coming from the background that you described. Still, are you sure you want to hear this?"

"Please, continue."

"You dedicate *Clayoquot* to Barbara Ellen but also to your 'wonderful mother.' Your mother may well have been wonderful, but when you write this, you are not fully aware of how angry you are with your own mother and how hurt you were by her. 'My mother was warm and loving, but I always knew she favoured my brother and sister. She was so full of love that some of it slopped over to me.' How does that actually feel to a child—whose perspective is this?"

"I never felt unloved."

"Of course you didn't feel unloved, and I'm not saying your mother didn't love you. But partially you didn't feel unloved because you shut off your pain around it. You write, 'After I grew up I once confronted my mother with my secret knowledge, and she was hurt and astonished and insisted that if she paid more attention to the other two, it was because they needed her more than I did, that I was always more emotionally independent.' That was your particular ruse to make it look like you are emotionally independent, to protect your mother and to avoid your hurt feelings. That was suppressing your own pain.

"'Although I always knew she favoured my brother and sister, she was so full of love some of it slopped over onto me' is also the perspective of an adult trying to distance herself from the emotional reality of the experience. The child's perspective would be different. How did it actually feel?"

"I know I used to resent the attention paid to my little sister because she would hold her breath and turn blue. Later, she studied to be a nurse practitioner, to get a nursing degree, and she had four children. She was an addict and an alcoholic, and she died before she was fifty from an overdose. My parents tried with her . . . my mother tried desperately with her."

"You're so quick to jump to your parents' defence."

"That's because I'm a parent."

"I think it's because you're defending yourself against your own pain in your relationship with your parents. You had nightmares . . . "

"Everybody would have nightmares if they drank all the iced tea I did . . ."

"Nightmares are about our deepest anxieties. A kid is afraid of monsters under the bed. You turn the light on and you show him that there are no monsters, and the next minute he is afraid of the monster again. What is he actually afraid of? He's afraid of not being protected, about not being connected enough. Maybe there's something monster-ish in the parent . . . maybe the parent is angry, so the kid is really scared. The kid has all this fear, so his mind will create the image of a monster."

"The nightmares I had were about my father. I detested him. Not too long ago, I was talking with my brother, who was very much browbeaten by my father. He became an aeronautical engineer in spite of all of it; although he himself has been a lifelong alcoholic, he's a functional one, and actually excels in his field. Not long ago he said, 'You know, Betty, I always admired you when we were kids because you weren't afraid to stand up to Dad.' That isn't true—I was petrified of Daddy, but I would offer some resistance. To my brother, in his mind, I was a freedom fighter because he would never say a single word to my father. My father called him a sissy because he just studied all the time."

"Another reason you had nightmares about him is that you couldn't talk to your mom about any of these feelings."

"What was I going to tell Mom—'I hate Daddy and I don't know what in the world you're doing with him'?"

"No, just 'Mom, I hate Daddy.'"

"It wouldn't have washed. The Bible says you honour your mother and father."

"I'm not blaming the mother because she is in this relationship—she has her own history. She can't very well fight and upset the applecart. But for the child, the bigger wound is the experience with the mother. You come from a mother's body and you relate to the mother. The mother is the universe for us. It's the universe that lets us down. When the father comes along as an abusive, threatening figure, the universe protects us or the universe doesn't protect us.

"Now, I'm not saying it's the mother's fault. It has to do with the position of women in society and the relationships people get into. I'm talking only about the child's experience. The child doesn't know it, since you can't miss what you're not familiar with, but the child is actually experiencing abandonment by the mom. When you say 'that wouldn't have washed,' what you're really saying is that your mother had no way of hearing your root feelings. We don't tend to think of that as wounding, but it is a deeper wound than anything else.

"There's a wonderful feminist book by Dorothy Dinnerstein, *The Mermaid and the Minotaur.* It discusses how the exclusive role that women have in early childraising distorts child development. When the woman is married to an immature man, she is also a mother to her husband, so she hasn't got the openness and the energy for her kids. So your real rival for your mother's affection wasn't your sister, it was your dad."

"It's so odd because all three of us before my sister died were talking one day about my father. The animosity that I feel for my father is nothing compared with what my sister and brother felt. They both hated my father so much. We were talking about my father, and my mother came into the room and she said, 'You know, when you kids talk about your father, I've always felt angry with you, because your father was a good man.' She also said, 'I don't think I paid enough attention to any of you. If I had it to do over again, I would pay more attention to all of you and less to Daddy.'"

"Perhaps. But she may not realize that he got the attention that he demanded. Had he had less, he would have made her suffer for it."

It was Barbara Ellen and her aunt who died of an overdose and her alcoholic uncle and her brave mother, Betty, and all Betty's children who, to one degree or another, suffered for the demanding immaturity of Betty's father and for the lack of true assertiveness by her mother. And these parents, too, were suffering and carrying the burden of generations. There is no one to blame, but there are generations on generations who had lived to bear a part in the genesis of Barbara Ellen's breast cancer.

7

Stress, Hormones,

Repression and Cancer

THE LARGE MAJORITY OF LUNG cancers are caused by carcinogens and tumour promoters ingested via cigarette smoking," says the twelfth edition of *Harrison's Principles of Internal Medicine*. The statement is scientifically incorrect, despite the truth it contains.

Smoking no more causes cancer of the lung than being thrown into deep water causes drowning. Fatal as immersion in deep water can be to the unprotected non-swimmer, for someone who swims well or is equipped with a life jacket, it poses little risk. A combination of factors is necessary to cause drowning. It is the same with lung cancer.

Smoking vastly increases the risk of cancer, not only of the lung but also of the bladder, the throat and other organs. But logic alone tells that us it cannot, by itself, *cause* any of these malignancies. If A causes B, then every time A is present, B should follow. If B does not follow A consistently, then A cannot, by itself, be the cause of B—even if, in most cases, it might be a major and perhaps necessary contributing factor. If smoking caused lung cancer, every smoker would develop the disease.

Several decades ago, David Kissen, a British chest surgeon, reported that patients with lung cancer were frequently characterized by a tendency to "bottle up" emotions.[1] In a number of studies, Kissen supported his clinical impressions that people with lung cancer "have poor and restricted outlets for the expression of emotion, as compared with non-malignancy lung patients and normal controls."[2] The risk of lung cancer, Kissen found, was five times higher in men who lacked the ability to express emotion effectively. Especially intriguing was that *those lung cancer patients who smoked but did not inhale exhibited even greater repression of emotion than those who did.* Kissen's observations implied that emotional repression works synergistically with smoking in the causation of lung cancer. The more severe the repression, the less the smoke damage required to result in cancer.

Kissen's insights were confirmed in spectacular fashion by a prospective study German, Dutch and Serbian researchers conducted over a ten-year period in Cvrenka, in the former Yugoslavia. The purpose of the study was to investigate the relationship of psychosocial risk factors to mortality. Cvrenka, an industrial town of about fourteen thousand inhabitants, was chosen partly because it was known to have a high mortality rate and partly because its stable population base permitted easier follow-up.

Nearly 10 per cent of the town's inhabitants were selected, about one thousand men and four hundred women. Each was interviewed in 1965–66, with a 109-item questionnaire that delineated such risk factors as adverse life events, a sense of long-lasting hopelessness and a hyper-rational, non-emotional coping style. Physical parameters like cholesterol levels, weight, blood pressure and smoking history were also recorded. People with already diagnosed disease were excluded from the research project.

By 1976, ten years later, over six hundred of the study participants had died of cancer, heart disease, stroke or other causes. The single greatest risk factor for death—and especially for cancer death—was what the researchers called rationality and anti-emotionality, or R/A. The eleven questions identifying R/A measured a single trait: the repression of anger. "Indeed *cancer incidence was some 40 times higher in those who answered positively to 10 or 11 of the questions for R/A than in the remaining subjects,* who answered positively to about 3 questions on average. . . .We found that smokers had no incidence of lung cancer unless they also had R/A scores of 10 or 11, *suggesting that any effect of smoking on the lung is essentially limited to a 'susceptible minority.'*"[3]

These findings do not absolve tobacco products or cigarette manufacturers of responsibility in the prevalence of lung cancer—on the contrary. All the thirty-eight people in the Cvrenka study who died of lung cancer had been smokers. The results indicated that for lung cancer to occur, tobacco alone is not enough: emotional repression must somehow potentiate the effects of smoke damage on the body. But how?

Psychological influences make a decisive biological contribution to the onset of malignant disease through the interconnections linking the components of the body's stress apparatus: the nerves, the hormonal glands, the immune system and the brain centres where emotions are perceived and processed.

Biologic and psychological activity are not independent; each represents the functioning of a super-system whose components can no longer be thought of as separate or autonomous mechanisms. The past quarter century of scientific inquiry has supplanted the traditional Western medical view of a split between body and mind with a truer, more unitary perspective. Candace Pert, a leading American researcher, has written that "the conceptual division between the sciences of immunology, endocrinology, and psychology/neuroscience is a historical artifact."[4] *Psychoneuroimmunology*—or, more comprehensively and accurately, *psychoneuroimmunoendocrinology*—is the name of the discipline that studies the interrelated functions of the organs and glands that regulate our behaviour and physiological balance.

The brain, nervous system, immune organs and immune cells and the endocrine glands are joined together through several pathways. As more research is done, more links are likely to be discovered. The combined task of this psychoneuroimmunoendocrine (PNI)* system is to ensure the development, survival and reproduction of each organism. The interconnections among the components of the PNI system enable it to recognize potential threats from within or without, and to respond with behaviours and biochemical changes coordinated to maximize safety at minimal cost.

The various parts of the PNI super-system are wired together by nervous system connections, some of them only recently identified. For example, the immune centres—previously thought of as acted on only by

---

* *The acronym PNI more commonly refers to the science of psychoneuroimmunoendocrinology.*
For convenience reasons I use it here to describe the physiological system that science studies: it is
tedious for both writer and reader to keep spelling out the word psychoneuroimmunoendocrine.

hormones—are extensively supplied with nerves. The so-called primary immune organs are the bone marrow and the thymus gland, located in the upper chest in front of the heart. Immune cells maturing in the bone marrow or in the thymus travel to the secondary lymph organs, including the spleen and the lymph glands. Fibres issuing from the central nervous system supply both primary and secondary lymph organs, allowing instant communication from the brain to the immune system. The hormone-producing endocrine glands are also directly wired to the central nervous system. Thus the brain can "talk" directly to the thyroid and adrenal glands, or to the testes and ovaries and other organs.

In turn, the hormones from the endocrine glands and substances produced by the immune cells directly affect brain activity. Chemicals from all these sources attach to receptors on the surfaces of brain cells, thereby influencing the organism's behaviour. We have all had the experience described in medical language as "sickness behaviour," which illustrates the action of immune products on the brain. A group of chemicals called cytokines, secreted by immune cells, can induce the feelings that prompt us to call in sick to our workplace—fever, loss of appetite, fatigue and increased need for sleep. Distressing as they are, such rapid adaptations are designed to conserve energy, helping us to overcome illness. Inappropriate secretion of the same substances, however, would interfere with normal functioning—for example, by causing excessive fatigue or chronic fatigue.

It is astonishing to learn that lymph cells and other white blood cells are capable of manufacturing nearly all the hormones and messenger substances produced in the brain and nervous system. Even endorphins, the body's intrinsic morphine-like mood-altering chemicals and painkillers, can be secreted by lymphocytes. And these immune cells also have on their surfaces receptors for the hormones and other molecules originating in the brain.

In short, in addition to the unifying network of nerve fibres that wire together the various components of the PNI super-system, there is also constant biochemical cross-talk among them. The myriad products they can each send to or receive from the others enable them all to speak and understand the same molecular language and to respond, each in its own way, to the same signals. The PNI system is like a giant switchboard, always alight with coordinated messages coming in from all directions and going out to all directions at the same time. It follows, too, that whatever short-term or chronic stimulus acts on any one part of the PNI system, it has the potential to affect the other parts as well.

What makes possible the versatile interactive functions of the PNI system? A microscopic look would reveal numerous receptor sites on the surface of each cell to which the common molecular messengers can bind. As Candace Pert reports, a typical nerve cell, or neuron, may have millions of receptors on its surface: "If you were to assign a different color to each of the receptors that scientists have identified, the average cell surface would appear as a multicolored mosaic of at least seventy different hues—50,000 of one type of receptor, 10,000 of another, 100,000 of a third, and so forth."[5]

The messenger molecules and most of the hormones are made of amino acids, the basic building blocks of protein. They are called peptides, the technical name for longer chains of amino acids. None of these chemicals are restricted to any one area or organ of the body. An eminent neuroscientist has suggested the term "information substances" to describe the entire group, because they each carry information from one cell or one organ to another. There are multiple potential interactions between information substances emanating from each part of the PNI system and cell types in each other part.

The hub of the PNI system is the hypothalamic-pituitary-adrenal nexus: the HPA axis. It is through the activation of the HPA axis that both psychological and physical stimuli set in motion the body's responses to threat. Psychological stimuli are first evaluated in the emotional centres known as the limbic system, which includes parts of the cerebral cortex and also deeper brain structures. If the brain interprets the incoming information as threatening, the hypothalamus will induce the pituitary to secrete an adrenocorticotropic hormone. ACTH, in turn, causes the cortex of the adrenal gland to secrete cortisol into the circulation.

Simultaneously with this hormonal cascade, the hypothalamus sends messages via the sympathetic nervous system—the flight-or-fight part of the nervous system—to another part of the adrenal, the medulla. The adrenal medulla manufactures and secretes the flight-fight hormone, adrenalin, which immediately stimulates the cardiovascular and nervous systems.

The same influences that the organism is most likely to interpret as emotionally stressful are, not surprisingly, also the most powerful psychic triggers for the HPA axis: "Psychological factors such as *uncertainty, conflict, lack of control, and lack of information* are considered the most stressful stimuli and strongly activate the HPA axis. Sense of control and consummatory behaviour result in immediate suppression of HPA activity."[6]

Consummatory behaviour—from the Latin *consummare,* "to complete"—is behaviour that removes the danger or relieves the tension caused by it. We recall that stress-inducing stimuli are not always objective external threats like predators or potential physical disasters but also include internal perceptions that something we consider essential is lacking. This is why lack of control, lack of information—and, as we will see, unsatisfied emotional needs (e.g., lack of love), trigger the HPA axis. Consummation of such needs abolishes the stress response.

Given the biochemical and neurological cross-influences within the PNI system, we can readily understand how emotions are able to interact with hormones, immune defences and the nervous system. In cancer causation, disturbed hormonal activity and impaired immune defences both play a role. Lung cancer is a prime example.

The mechanistic view holds that cancer results from damage to the DNA of a cell by some noxious substance—for example, tobacco-breakdown products. This perspective is valid as far it goes but cannot explain why some smokers develop cancers while others do not, even if the amount and type of tobacco they inhale are exactly the same. The unanswered questions are, Why are the cells of some individuals more susceptible than those of others? Why does DNA repair occur in some people but not in others? Why do the immune system and other defences keep cancer at bay in some people but not in others? What accounts for vast differences in cure or disease progression from one person to the next, even when the identical cancer is diagnosed at exactly the same stage and even when all other factors—age, gender, income, general health—are exactly matched?

Genetic variations may explain these issues in some cancers, although, as we have seen with breast cancer, in the majority of people heredity does not play a role in cancer causation. Lung cancer, specifically, is not a genetically transmitted disease, nor is the damage to genes in lung cancer due to heredity.

The development of any malignancy progresses through several stages, the first of which is *initiation,* the process by which a normal cell becomes transformed into an abnormal one. Cancer may be seen as a disease of cell replication. The normal processes of cell division and cell death are somehow subverted. A cell that should give rise to healthy offspring escapes from control and divides into malformed facsimiles that replicate themselves without regard to the biological needs of the organism. With millions of cells dying or being formed in the body every day, natural accident would, by itself, lead to a great number of spontaneous abnormal transformations. "It's a fact that every one of us has a number of tiny cancerous tumours growing in our bodies at every moment," writes Candace Pert.

Tobacco smoke has a directly damaging effect on the genetic material of lung cells. It has been estimated that for the initiation of cancer, lung cells have to acquire as many as ten separate lesions or points of damage on their DNA. Yet, no matter where in the body, such genomic damage "seldom leads to tumour formation. This is principally due to the fact that most primary lesions are transient and are readily eliminated by DNA repair or cell death."[7] In other words, DNA repairs itself or the cell dies without replicating its damaged genetic material—which, no doubt, accounts for the fact that most smokers do not develop clinical lung cancer. Where cancer does arise, either DNA repair or the normal process of cell death must have failed. In a 1999 review of psychological effects on lung cancer, researchers from the Ohio State University College of Medicine wrote: "Faulty DNA repair is associated with an increased incidence of cancer. Stress may alter these DNA repair mechanisms; for example, in one study, lymphocytes from psychiatric inpatients with higher depressive symptoms demonstrated impairment in their ability to repair cellular DNA damaged by exposure to X-irradiation [X-rays]."[8] Impaired DNA repair has also been documented in studies of stressed laboratory animals.

Apoptosis is the scientific term for the physiologically regulated death necessary for the maintenance of healthy tissues. Apoptosis ensures normal tissue turnover, culling older cells with weakened genetic material, leaving room for their healthy and vigorous offspring. "Dysregulated apoptosis contributes to many pathologies, including tumour production, autoimmune and immunodeficiency diseases, and neurodegenerative disorders."[9]

Steroid hormones released through the activity of the HPA axis help regulate apoptosis in a number of ways. Habitual repression of emotion leaves a person in a situation of chronic stress, and chronic stress creates an unnatural biochemical milieu in the body. Perpetually abnormal steroid hormone levels can interfere with normal programmed cell death. Also participating in cell death are natural killer cells. Depression—a mental state in which repression of anger dominates emotional functioning—interacts with cigarette smoking to lower the activity of NK cells.[10]

In short, for cancer causation it is not enough that DNA damage occur: also necessary are failure of DNA repair and/or an impairment of regulated cell death. Stress and the repression of emotion can negatively affect both of those processes. The findings of the Cvrenka investigators and of the British surgeon David Kissen make physiological sense when we consider the first stage of malignant transformation, that of initiation.

A two-part article published in the *Canadian Medical Association Journal* in 1996 reviewed the role of the PNI system in health and disease. "In healthy people," noted the authors, "neuroimmune mechanisms provide host defence against infection, injury, cancer, and control immune and inflammatory reactions, which pre-empt disease."[11] Disease, in other words, is not a simple result of some external attack but develops in a vulnerable host in whom the internal environment has become disordered.

Subsequent phases of cancerous change are *promotion* and *progression*. Having escaped the normal regulatory mechanisms that should have prevented their survival, the newly malignant cells continue to divide, leading to the formation of a tumour. At this stage, tumour growth can be inhibited or supported by the body's internal environment. The PNI super-system comes into play. Acting chiefly through hormonal regulation by the HPA axis, it creates a milieu in the body tissues that is either receptive or hostile to the growth and spread of cancer.

"The chronic psychological status of the individual may play an important role either in facilitating tumour promotion or in dampening or accentuating the impacts of environmental stress," Dr. Marc E. Lippman, head of the breast cancer section, Medicine Branch, National Cancer Institute, Bethesda, Maryland, has written. "The human endocrine system

provides one critical mediator of interaction between psyche and tumor.
. . . It seems inescapable that psychic factors which can evoke endocrine
changes will have effects on actual tumour biology."[12]

The effect of hormones on the growth and spread of cancer is
twofold. First, many tumours are directly hormone dependent, or they
arise in organs intimately involved in hormonal interactions, such as
the ovaries or the testes. Hormone-dependent cancer cells bear on
their membranes receptors for various hormones capable of promoting
cell growth. One example of a hormone-dependent cancer is that of the
breast. It is generally understood that many breast cancers are estrogen dependent, this being the rationale for the use of the estrogen-blocking drug
tamoxifen. Less well known is that some breast cancers have receptors
for a broad array of other "information substances," including androgens
(male sex hormones), progestins, prolactin, insulin, vitamin D and several
more—all of them secreted by the HPA axis or regulated by it.

Stress is a powerful modulator of hormonal function, as seen in both
human experience and animal studies. In one experiment, researchers
manipulated the dominance relationships in groups of female monkeys.
Established dominance patterns were broken up. Some previously dominant animals were forced into subordination, while subordinate ones
were enabled to achieve dominant status.

Social subordination caused hormonal dysfunctions of the HPA axis
and of the ovaries. "Females that were currently dominant secreted less
cortisol than those who were currently subordinate." Dominant female
monkeys had normal menstruations and higher concentrations of proges-
terone prior to ovulation. Subordinates ovulated less often and more
frequently had impaired menstrual cycles.

When the experimental situation was altered so that previously
dominant monkeys became subordinate, their reproductive function
was almost immediately suppressed and their cortisol production went
up. The reverse was the case in monkeys previously subordinate but
newly made dominant.[13]

Cancers of the female gynecological organs such as the ovaries and
the uterus are also hormone related. Ovarian malignancy is only the
seventh most common cancer in women, but it is the fourth leading
cause of cancer deaths. Of all cancers, it carries the highest tumour-
to-death ratio: that is, it has the poorest prognosis. In 1999, twenty-six

hundred Canadian women were diagnosed with ovarian cancer. In the same year, fifteen hundred died of it. In the U.S. about twenty thousand women are diagnosed annually; nearly two-thirds of them will succumb to the disease. Although early treatment is highly effective, by the time most cases are diagnosed, the cancer has advanced beyond the ability of current treatment to cure it.

As yet there are no effective screening tests to identify the initial stages of this disease. Ultrasounds and a blood test, called CA-125, are useful in monitoring treatment, but neither is reliable as a tool to find the cancer before it causes symptoms or before it spreads beyond its site of origin. Darlene, an insurance broker, was diagnosed during the course of an infertility workup. "They did a laparoscopy to look at my ovaries," she says, "and that's how they found the cancer. So instead of a child, I ended up with an oophorectomy."

Since infertility is one of the known risk indicators for ovarian cancer, hormonal factors are obviously important. Unfortunately, the picture is confusing. Early menses and late menopause increase the risk of developing ovarian cancer, while pregnancies and the birth control pill decrease it. This pattern would suggest that the more women ovulate, the more susceptible they become to the disease. On the other hand, infertility—when no ovulation takes place—also adds to the risk. Evidently the hormonal influences here are subtle and complicated. What we do know about the hormones of female reproduction is that they are exquisitively sensitive to women's psychological states and to the stresses in their lives. Hormonal function may also be related to certain character traits, as a study at the University of Pittsburgh in 2001 concluded.

Researchers at the Pittsburgh School of Medicine compared the psychological characterisitics of women with chronically missed periods—amenorrhea—with women whose menstruation was normal. They were particularly interested in a group with functional hypothalamic amenorrhea (FHA), that is, the group of women who had no identifiable disease or condition to account for the lack of normal ovulation. The study found that "the women with FHA reported more dysfunctional attitudes, particularly those associated with need for approval. [They] were more likely . . . to endorse attitudes that are prevalent among persons vulnerable to depression, such as perfectionistic standards and concern about the judgment of others.[14]

A major finding of the Pittsburgh researchers was the discovery of subtly but significantly disturbed eating habits in non-menstruating women. Troubled eating patterns are inextricably linked with unresolved childhood issues, as we will see, for example, in the case of the comedienne Gilda Radner who died of ovarian cancer. The stresses that create the problems with self-nurture are also stresses that predispose to ill health. The authors of the Pittsburgh study write that "women with FHA report more concerns about dieting and weight, fear of weight gain, and tendencies to engage in binge eating."

Eating patterns are directly connected with emotional issues arising both from childhood and from current stresses. The patterns of how we eat or don't eat, and how much we eat, are strongly related to the levels of stress we experience and to the coping responses we have developed in face of life's vicissitudes. In turn, dietary habits intimately affect the functioning of the hormones that influence the female reproductive tract. Anorexics, for example, will often stop menstruating.

Jerilynn Prior, a Vancouver endocrinologist with a special interest in women's health issues, found that subtle hormonal disruptions can occur even among women who report regular periods and no symptoms. She wrote in the *Canadian Journal of Diagnosis:* "Approximately one-third of regular, asymptomatic menstrual cycles of healthy women will have disturbances of ovulation that, based on biologic principles, could lead to significant health risks."[15]

The commonest cause of failed ovulation in Dr. Prior's study was insufficient stimulation of the ovaries by the hypothalamus and pituitary due to "an imbalance or incoordination in the signals sent from the hypothalamus and pituitary gland to the ovarian follicle." These disturbances, wrote Dr. Prior, "are caused by adaptions related to life cycle, changes in weight, psychosocial stresses, excessive exercise, or illness."

Malignancies of the hematological (blood-cell producing) system such as leukemia and lymphoma are also hormone dependent, being profoundly affected by cortisol produced in the adrenal gland. Adrenal corticoid hormones inhibit the division and spread of leukemia and lymphoma cells. Thus, hematological malignancies may, in part, result when blood and lymph cells escape from normal inhibition owing to a chronically unbalanced HPA system. The available research points to emotional stress as a significant dynamic in the lives of adults with these diseases.

At the University of Rochester, a fifteen-year study of people who developed lymphoma or leukemia reportedly found that these malignancies were "apt to occur in a setting of emotional loss or separation which in turn brought about feelings of anxiety, sadness, anger or hopelessness."[16]

Synthetic analogues of the stress hormone cortisol are important components of the treatment of leukemia and lymphoma. Interestingly, the amount of cortisol-like hormone needed to block the replication of leukemic cells is only a little higher than what should normally be functionally available in the body. In the case of leukemia, episodes of acute stress in which the cortisol levels temporarily rise are sometimes enough to induce a remission. Such is thought to have happened during the illness of the composer Béla Bartók.

We need to recall here that the temporary elevation of cortisol that occurs in episodes of *acute* stress is healthy and necessary. Not healthy are the chronically elevated cortisol levels in chronically stressed persons.

Bartók, in exile from his native Hungary and stricken with leukemia, was commissioned by the conductor of the Boston Symphony Orchestra, Serge Koussevitsky, to write a new piece. The composer went into spontanous remission, which lasted until the work was completed. Quite likely, HPA-triggered cortisol and several other elements of the PNI system contributed to this famous remission, which made possible the creation of Bartók's *Concerto for Orchestra,* a classic of twentieth-century music.

Apart from their direct effects on hormone-dependent malignancies, hormones regulated by the stress-sensitive HPA axis and by limbic areas of the brain act on other tissues in the body to influence the development of cancers. Chief among these hormone-sensitive tissues is the immune system.

It is customary to conceive of cancer as an invader against whom the body—like a country under foreign attack—must wage war. Such a view, while perhaps comforting in its simplicity, is a distortion of reality. First, even when there is an external carcinogen like tobacco, the cancer itself is partially an outcome of internal processes gone wrong. And, of course, for most cancers there is no such identified carcinogen. Second, it is the internal environment, locally and throughout the entire organism, that plays the major role in deciding whether the malignancy will flourish or be eliminated. The malignant transformation of normal cells, in other words, is a process determined by many factors that have at least as much to do with the biopsychosocial state of the organism as with the type of cancer itself.

Once a cancer reaches the stage where its cell surfaces display molecules different from the normal body proteins, it ought to be destroyed by immune responses of many different kinds. T-cells should attack it with noxious chemicals; antibodies should be formed against it; specialized blood cells should chew it up. Under conditions of chronic stress, the immune system may become either too confused to recognize the mutated cell clones that form the cancer or too debilitated to mount an effective attack against them.

Also implicated in the growth and development of tumours are a large number of locally produced chemicals, some secreted by the cancer cells themselves. Such chemicals include growth factors, inhibitory substances and messenger molecules of many kinds. A complicated balance among them will tilt the process toward either tumour suppression or tumour growth. Suffice it to say here that this intricate biochemical cascade is profoundly influenced by the PNI system, particularly through hormones and other information substances.

Finally, emotional states are of great potential significance in the prevention or encouragement of cancer metastasis, the movement of malignant cells from the original tumour site to other areas of the body.

In popular mythology, cancer has to be "caught early" before it has a chance to spread. The biological reality is quite different: by the time a tumour becomes detectable, spread has, in many cases, already occurred. "A high proportion of early cancers have already thrown off occult metastases by the time the primary tumour is diagnosed," the British oncologist Basil Stoll has pointed out.[17] However, most metastases either die or lie dormant for a long time.

Doubling time—the amount of time needed for a tumour mass to double in size—varies from one cancer type to another, and there are great variations within individual cancer types. For a tumour to become clinically noticeable, even on an easily accessible body tissue like the skin or the breast, it has to become about half a gram in size, comprising about five hundred million cells. A single cell with a malignant mutation would have to double about thirty times to reach such dimensions.[18] In breast cancer, doubling time has been calculated to range from a few days to one and one-half years, with an average of about four months. "If a tumour cell were to grow constantly at the last rate, it would take about eight years to become clinically evident, and some sources suggest an even longer doubling time with a time span of about 15–20 years to become clinically evident."[19]

In the real life of a tumour, there is probably no steady doubling rate. Rather, there are broad fluctuations in growth rate depending on what is happening in the life of the host. We recall the history of Michelle, whose breast lump, which had been present for seven years, changed dramatically after a period of acute stress.

Since breast cancers have the potential to metastasize by the time they are a little over half a millimetre in diameter, "if a tumor is going to metastasize, in general it will already have done so by the time [it] is clinically detectable."[20] Microscopic spread of malignant cells seems to happen in many cases of breast cancer without ever causing clinical problems. In other cases, the metastatic deposit may lie dormant in distant tissues for years and then, unexpectedly, declare itself in the form of symptoms. The same dynamic operates with prostate cancer, which is why spread has already occurred in 40 per cent of prostate malignancies by the time the diagnosis is made. In fact, in a striking similarity with prostate cancer, autopsy studies on women indicate that as many as 25 to 30 per cent of all women have microscopic breast malignancies, "far in excess of the number ever actually manifested."[21]

The issue, therefore, is not simply the prevention of spread, but why and under what conditions in some people already existing dormant deposits convert into clinical cancer. Tumour dormancy is affected by many hormonal and immunological influences, all of them functions of the PNI system and all of them highly susceptible to life stresses.

There are dramatic fluctuations in tumour growth rates from one patient to the next. Also evident is a high degree of inconsistency in the appearance of metastatic disease and of survival times among patients who, clinically, are diagnosed with exactly the same type of cancer at the same stage of severity. For example, there are "many cases where incompletely excised breast cancers never recur, or where secondary deposits lie dormant in the host tissues for up to 30 years before finally manifesting."[22] Such individual differences, it would seem, are due not to the autonomous behaviour of the malignancy but to factors in the body's internal environment that inhibit the growth of cancer or, conversely, encourage it. That internal milieu is profoundly affected by the stressors acting on people's lives and also by the highly variable ways in which individuals cope with stress.

In numerous studies of cancer, the most consistently identified risk factor is the inability to express emotion, particularly the feelings associated with anger. The repression of anger is not an abstract emotional trait that mysteriously leads to disease. It is a major risk factor because it increases physiological stress on the organism. It does not act alone but in conjunction with other risk factors that are likely to accompany it, such as hopelessness and lack of social support. The person who does not feel or express "negative" emotion will be isolated even if surrounded by friends, because his real self is not seen. The sense of hopelessness follows from the chronic inability to be true to oneself on the deepest level. And hopelessness leads to helplessness, since nothing one can do is perceived as making any difference.

One study dealt with healthy women who had no symptoms, only an abnormal Pap smear on a routine physical examination. Without any knowledge of the results of the Pap smear, the researchers "were able to predict with almost 75 per cent accuracy those individuals who had early cancer, simply by utilizing a questionnaire which differentiated between various emotional states. They found that cancer was most apt to occur in those women with a 'helplessness–prone personality,' or some sense of helpless frustration which could not be resolved in the preceding six months."[23]

The researchers in Cvrenka had also predicted who among their nearly fourteen hundred subjects would likely develop cancer and die of it, based on the psychological characteristics of rationality/anti-emotionality (repressed anger) and a long-lasting sense of hopelessness. When they checked the death records ten years later, they found they had been right in 78 per cent of cases. "It seems to us," they commented, "that the importance of psychosomatic risk factors is likely to have been grossly underestimated in many studies."

The influence of psychological risk factors is poignantly illustrated in

the life history of Gilda Radner. Radner's maternal aunt and two cous-
ins died of ovarian cancer, and her mother was successfully treated for
breast cancer. Gilda faced a genetic risk, but was she absolutely fated to
die of ovarian cancer? There is no reason to think so.

For most women who develop ovarian cancer, heredity does not
figure heavily among the risk factors. For a few, it is highly significant.
About 8 per cent of women with ovarian cancer carry one of the
genetic mutations known to increase risk. In fact, these are the same
BRCA genes implicated in breast cancer. Depending on which strand
of DNA is involved, those with the mutation in one gene could have
a 63 per cent risk of developing cancer by age seventy. Those women
whose mutation is in the other gene have a 27 per cent risk of ovarian
cancer by age seventy-five.[24] For women without the mutation but who
have a first-degree relative—mother, sister or daughter—with ovarian
cancer, the risk is about 5 per cent. Here again, we see that genes by
themselves do not tell the whole story. Even in these high-risk categories, not everyone is ordained to develop cancer.

Gilda Radner sparkled with manic energy and a zest for experience, but she carried the psychological burdens of a highly stressful and
self-negating life. The eating disorder she suffered from likely affected
her hormonal balance. She was also infertile, due probably to the type
of hypothalamic-pituitary dysfunction discussed earlier in this chapter.

The slim star of *Saturday Night Live* was bulimic. By her own
description, she had been an "unhappy, fat and mediocre" child. She
characterized her childhood as a "nightmare." "My brother and I ate
ourselves into little balloon children," she wrote in her memoir. "We
looked like no-neck monsters. My parents sent me to summer camp
every year and every year I was scapegoated. . . . In the 'princess game'
there would be controlling girls and pretty girls. The controlling girls
would make the pretty girl the princess, and the controlling girls would
be the advisors to the princess. The fat girl would be the servant or
something, and that would be me."[25]

Gilda's relationship with her mother appears to have been intensely
negative, and apparently marked by competition for her father's attention. Gilda maintained that her father had been "the love of my life."
His death of brain cancer, when she was twelve, was an irreparable loss.

All her adult life, Gilda, out of sheer desperation, promiscuously sought male love and acceptance. "To a great extent my life has been controlled by the men I loved," she wrote. She attempted to make herself into whatever woman she thought the man in her life preferred.

Gilda found it impossible to speak her emotional truth to her mother, Henrietta, or to say no to her directly. When already a star and a closet bulimic, she would attempt to allay her mother's anxieties about what she ate by concocting detailed fabrications of imaginary meals. Henrietta did not learn about her daughter's bulimia while Gilda was alive.

Using comedy, Gilda could control her environment. Comedy filled a crucial childhood need. It was a way of endearing herself to her father and her sole means of reaching her mother, "a way of getting to her when nothing worked." She became a "natural" comic. The price was the obliteration of her own feelings.

Gilda was a self-confessed workaholic who, she would write, "let stress and pressure run my precious life." On a youthful trip to Paris, she threw herself in front of traffic in a dramatic suicidal gesture that could easily have killed her. "At least someone cares about me," she said to the friend who pulled her to safety.

Even after her symptoms of ovarian cancer began to cause physical distress, including bowel blockage, Radner was more concerned with satisfying others than with her own needs. She sought and received advice from sundry sources. Her dilemma? "Suddenly I began to wonder how to please so many people. Do I take magnesium citrate? What about the coffee enema? Do I do both? Do I do the abdominal massage or the colonic? Do I tell the doctors about each other? East meets West in Gilda's body: Western medicine down my throat, Eastern medicine up my butt."

When it seemed she had been successfully treated, Gilda became a poster girl for ovarian cancer, featured on the cover of *Life* magazine. She was an inspiration to many, but the recovery was short-lived. Still attached to roles she had developed as a child, she berated herself for having "let down" others by developing terminal illness. "I had become a spokeswoman for The Wellness Community, and a symbol of getting well. I had been a model cancer patient completely active in my own therapy. Now

I felt like a living example that didn't work. *I'm just a fraud,** I thought."

Only close to her death did Gilda finally learn that she could not be mother to the world. "I couldn't do everything I wanted to do. I couldn't keep calling all the cancer patients I knew, and I couldn't try to help heal all the women with ovarian cancer, and I couldn't read every letter I received because it was ripping me apart. . . . I couldn't cry all those tears for everybody else, I had to take care of myself. . . . It is important to realize that you have to take care of yourself because you can't take care of anybody else until you do."

---

* *Radner's italics.*

8

Something Good

Comes Out of This

E D WAS DIAGNOSED AFTER HIS general practicioner found a small nodule during a routine rectal exam. "I went for a biopsy," he reports, "and they did six hits on the prostate. They found an irregularity in one hit. Prostate cancer. Since then I've looked at all the options, and it was all either slash, burn or poison. I've spoken with a lot of men who have had their prostate removed, and some who have had radiation. It's been pretty lousy for most of them."

"You haven't had any medical treatment?" I ask Ed.

"I've been to a naturopath, and I am doing hypnotherapy, and I've been doing a lot of looking at myself and how I've lived my life."

Ed's colourful phrase, "slash, burn or poison" refers to the three major types of treatment currently offered for prostate cancer: surgery, radiation and chemotherapy. Although some patients come through such treatments without harm, others suffer unpleasant consequences such as urinary incontinence and impotence. A review of over a hundred thousand prostatectomy cases published in 1999 concluded that "complications and re-admission after prostatectomy are substantially more common than previously recognized."[1]

Those risks might be acceptable if the treatments available cured disease or saved lives, but the evidence is ambivalent at best. The loud public campaigns urging men to undergo screening tests for prostate cancer by means of the rectal digital exam or the prostate specific antigen (PSA) blood tests have no proven scientific basis. "I think it's important for people to realize that once we find their prostate cancer, we still have no evidence that treatment works," Timothy Wilt, associate professor of medicine at the Minneapolis Veterans Affairs Medical Center, told *The New York Times*.[2] "And that's really the whole crux of the screening issue: If treatment doesn't work, why are we using the PSA to look for tumors?"

Supporters of aggressive medical approaches ought to be disheartened by statistics gathered by Dr. Otis Brawley, a medical oncologist and epidemiologist at the U.S. National Cancer Institute. In places where screening is widely practiced, the incidence of diagnosed prostate cancer goes up, and the number of men being treated increases, but the death rate from prostatic malignancy remains unchanged.[3] If anything, prostate cancer mortality rates were slightly higher in the intensely screened areas. Also disturbing are findings published in *The Journal of the National Cancer Institute,* that men aggressively treated for prostate cancer had a higher chance of dying of other cancers than men who did not receive any medical intervention.[4]

Although some prostate cancer probably should receive treatment, at this point it is not known exactly who would benefit from intervention. Most prostate cancers are very slow to develop, so much so that the man is likely to die before the malignancy triggers any health problems, if it ever would. In others cases, the cancer is so aggressive that by the time of diagnosis, treatment makes no difference. Since there is no reliable way of deciding when treatment works, what are people who "survive" their prostate cancer really surviving—their treatment or their disease? In the case of prostate malignancy, medicine as it is commonly practised simply does not apply the usual scientific standards.

Public opinion is based on the common-sense view that the sooner a condition is discovered, the more likely doctors will be able to cure it. Convinced that medical intervention saved their lives, celebrities like Gen. Norman Schwarzkopf, the golfer Arnold Palmer or the Canadian federal cabinet minister Allan Rock—all diagnosed with prostate cancer after screening tests—act as persuasive advocates of early diagnosis. Men need to let science, not the latest public figure endorsing PSA testing, help them make a decision about prostate cancer screening and treatment, Dr. Otis Brawley told *The Journal of the American Medical Association*.[5]

Despite scientific confusion, bias toward treatment is powerful. Few doctors are willing to let nature take its course in the face of potential disease, even if the value of intervention is questionable. And men, even if well informed, may choose to "do something" rather than tolerate the anxiety of inaction. But patients always deserve to be told what is known about prostate cancer—and, just as important, all that remains unknown.

Prostate cancer was the first human malignancy to be linked with hormonal influences. Just as cancer of the breast may improve in women who have their ovaries removed, so castration leads to a shrinking of prostate tumours, due to diminished levels of androgens, or male hormones. Orchidectomy, the surgical removal of the testicles, remains part of the treatment arsenal, as does the adminstration of powerful medications blocking the effects of the male hormones. Such "chemical castration" is the first-line treatment now offered men with metastatic prostate cancer.

Given the strong connection between hormone levels and emotions, it is striking how completely medical research and medical practice have ignored psychological influences on the causation of prostate cancer and have eschewed more holistic approaches to its treatment. There has been virtually no investigation of personality or stress factors in prostate malignancy. Textbooks ignore the subject.

The neglect of potential links between stress, emotions and prostate cancer is all the less justifiable given what is already known. By their thirties, many men will have some cancerous cells in their prostate, and by their eighties, the majority are found to have them. By the age of fifty, a man has a 42 per cent chance of developing prostate cancer. Yet relatively few men at any age will progress to the point of overt clinical disease. In other words, the presence of cancerous prostate cells is not unusual even in younger men, and it becomes the norm as men get older. Only in a minority does it progress to the formation of a tumour that causes symptoms or threatens life. It is worth asking how stress may promote the development of malignant disease. What personality patterns or life circumstances may interfere with the body's defence mechanisms, allowing the already-present cancer cells to proliferate?

As I arrived to interview Ed, a wiry man with a body and face of someone years younger than his age of forty-four, he turned to his wife, Jean, who was just leaving to go shopping. "It's a pain in the ass," he said, "but I have to go and look at so-and-so's truck for him. It's not starting."

"Let me ask you something right away," I begin.

"Sure."

"You're saying that looking at this guy's truck is a pain in the ass. Now that's an interesting metaphor, anatomically, when used by somebody who has cancer of the prostate. How easy has it been in your life to say no to things that were actually more of a pain in the ass than a benefit to you?"

"I really don't say no. I try to help people all the time."

"Even if it's a pain?"

"Yeah. Even if it's not the greatest time for me, or I should be doing other things that are more important for me. I like to help people out."

"What happens if you don't?"

"I feel bad about it. Guilty."

Ed, leader of a country music band, used to do cocaine, mescaline and marijuana, "two or three joints a day, my whole youth. A problem for me ever since my childhood has been alcohol." Ed tells me about his first adult relationship, which lasted ten years. He lived with an older woman whose two children he helped to bring up, drinking daily to suppress his unhappiness. That relationship came to an end when his partner had an affair.

"I threw in the towel. I said, I don't want to put up with this. I never screwed around, even though I felt like it. From that day on, I quit drinking for a year and a half, started jogging and doing what I wanted to do. I had this free feeling, like this huge weight was off my chest. I could do anything I wanted to and I felt so good about myself."

"How much are you drinking these days?"

"Maybe about four beer a day. Every day."

"What does it do for you?"

"Jean and I got hooked up, and her problems become my problems, and it just gets heavier and heavier and heavier, and then I start with alcohol again."

"So in some ways you are not happy in this marriage."

"I guess the biggest thing is the control factor. I've allowed Jean to take control of this marriage, because of her multiple sclerosis and because she came from such an abusive marriage.* She was dictated to,

---

* Jean has MS. For her story, see chapter 18, "The Power of Negative Thinking."

told what clothes to wear and all that kind of stuff. What in turn it's done is made me cower in this marriage."

"So you see yourself as being controlled. How do you feel about that?"

"I'm resentful."

"And how do you deal with it?"

"I hide it."

"You don't tell her that you don't like it?"

"No. I don't."

"What does that remind you of?"

"My childhood? Exactly."

Although Ed had told me previously that he had had a "very great upbringing," it soon became evident that he had felt controlled by his parents and full of guilt if he failed to meet their expectations. He recalled he had received what he called "deserved spankings," which, on further inquiry, turned out to have been beatings with a belt administered by his father, from about age eight on. "He believed that that was the best way of doing things."

"What do you believe?"

"Well, now, I don't think that was the best thing he could do, but you really don't have much choice when you're a young child. I wanted to be a good person. When you're a child looking at your father, you don't know what he's supposed to be, because you want your dad to be perfect, and you want to be a perfect child."

One of the puzzling features of prostate malignancy is that while testosterone—the hormone people have been led to believe is responsible for male aggression—seems to promote its growth, this cancer is most typically a disease of older men. Yet the body's production of testosterone declines with aging. Nor have men with prostate cancer been shown to have higher than average blood levels of testosterone. As with estrogen receptors in breast cancer, it appears the sensitivity of tumour cells to normal concentrations of testosterone must have been altered.

Like hormone secretion by the adrenal glands and the ovaries, the synthesis of testosterone by the testicles is under the complex feedback control of the hypothalamic–pituitary system in the brain. That network, highly reactive to stress and emotions, sends a cascade of biological substances into circulation. Emotional factors can directly influence male sex-hormone functioning for good or ill—just as the female hormone estrogen from the ovaries, or adrenalin, cortisol and other hormones from the adrenal glands, are affected by psychic events. It so happens that in a small series of patients, surgical removal of the brain's pituitary gland did show positive results in the treatment of prostate cancer.[6]

Testosterone gets a bad rap. If one wishes to compliment a woman's self-confidence or assertiveness, one will assert that she "has balls." A Canadian columnist wrote in praise of Margaret Thatcher, the iron-willed—or merciless, depending on one's vantage point—former British prime minister, that she had "10 times more testosterone than the men." Meanwhile, male destructiveness and hostile aggression are frequently blamed on testosterone. In actual fact, high levels of the hormone are more an effect than a cause.

Victory or defeat was shown to alter not only the hormonal balance but even the brain cells in a species of fish, the African cichlid. "In defeat, the fish's hypothalamic cells shrink with consequent declines in reproductive hormones and shrinkage of the testes." If the situation is manipulated to permit defeated fish to become dominant, there is a dramatic growth of the cells in the hypothalamus that produce a gonadotropin-releasing hormone (GRH), which stimulates the pituitary to produce hormones that act on the testes. The testes, in turn, will now increase in size, and the fish's sperm counts will improve. "Most importantly, this research has clearly demonstrated . . . *that it is the behavioural changes* [i.e., the attainment of dominant status] *that lead to the subsequent physiologic changes.*"[7]

As highly evolved creatures, we may like to believe that our gonadal functioning is not as readily susceptible to life's ups and downs as that of the lowly African cichlid. In fact, human hormone levels, like those in our African fish, may follow rather than precede changes in dominance relationships. Prof. James Dabbs, a social psychologist at Georgia State University in Atlanta, has researched the interaction of testosterone and behaviour. According to a report in *The New York Times,* after reviewing his nearly forty studies he has concluded that while testosterone does increase libido, "there is no proof it causes aggression." On the other hand, there is proof that emotional states can rapidly alter testosterone production: "Dr. Dabbs tested fans before and immediately after the 1994 World Cup of soccer final between Italy and Brazil. In what Dr. Dabbs considers proof of the axiom 'basking in reflected glory,' testosterone levels swelled among the victorious Brazilians and sank among the dejected Italians."[8] Not surprisingly, then, gonadal function is affected by psychological states in both men and women. In depressed men, the secretion of testosterone and other hormones connected with sexual functioning were found to be significantly diminished.[9] A hormone-dependent malignancy like that of the prostate may be highly susceptible to biochemical influences related to stress and emotional states.

Cancer of the prostate is the second commonest malignancy of men. Only cancer of the lung occurs more frequently. Calculations vary, but in the United States in 1996 as many as 317,000 new cases were estimated, and about 41,000 deaths.[10] About 20,000 new cases are diagnosed in Canada each year.

Environmental factors must be significant. Japanese men migrating to Hawaii and the continental United States were found to have a higher incidence of the disease than those natives of the country who stayed in Japan: over two and a half times as great. Yet on autopsies of men without clinical disease, similar rates of inactive malignant cells were found regardless of geography.[11] The question, then, is, Why do these inactive cells develop into cancerous tumours in one environment but not in another? There are highly suggestive epidemiological findings to indicate that stress crucially influences who will and who will not suffer illness and death from prostate cancer.

Family history increases the risk for prostate cancer, but it is not a major factor in most instances. No specific cancer-inducing environmental agents have been identified comparable to, say, cigarettes and lung cancer. Saturated fats may play a role. Given the wide geographic variation, so may genetic influences. The disease is most prevalent in the Scandinavian countries, least in Asia. The single racial/ethnic group at highest risk in the world are African Americans, among whom prostate cancer is twice as common as among the U.S. white population.

"African-American men have a poorer survival rate than whites for all stages of prostate cancer when the cancer is diagnosed at younger ages."[12] One could ascribe this higher death rate to the reduced access to medical care generally available to lower-middle-class and working-class people in the U.S. health system. However, the racial differences in prostate malignancy cut across class lines. In any case, greater access to medical care has not so far been shown to have any positive effect on survival. We could possibly attempt to explain the difference in death rates by referring to genetic factors, except that American blacks experience prostate cancer at a sixfold rate compared with black men in Nigeria. Here, too, the presence of clinically "silent" prostate cancer cells is the same in the two groups.[13]

Now, if environmental factors such as caloric intake were responsible for the development of the disease, one would not expect much difference in the death rate between American whites and blacks. As it stands, only about 10 per cent of the black/white variation in cancer rate has been estimated to be due to the intake of saturated fats.[14] If, on the other hand, genetic influences were decisive, disease rates between blacks in the U.S. and Nigeria ought to be much closer than they are.

The historical, social and economic position of black people in U.S. society has undermined cohesion in black communities and black families and has imposed greater psychological stress on African Americans than their Caucasian fellow citizens or that blacks in Africa find themselves under. There is a parallel here in the higher occurrence of elevated blood pressure among American blacks. Hypertension is a condition clearly related to stress. In an analogous example, the rates of an autoimmune disease, rheumatoid arthritis, suffered by blacks in South Africa under apartheid increased as they migrated to the city from their native villages, even if in strict financial terms they may have gained by the move. The major factor would seem to be the psychological pressures of living in an environment where official racism directly and overtly deprived people of autonomy and dignity, while it uprooted people from their traditional family and social supports.

A finding consistent with what we have seen elsewhere in relationship to disease and emotional isolation is that men who are currently married, compared with men who are divorced or widowed, are less likely to be diagnosed with prostate cancer.[15] While I was not able to find in the literature any other investigation specific to prostate cancer and psychological factors, one study did look at men who had greater dependency needs than a comparable group—that is, men who were less able to experience themselves as individuated, self-reliant adults.

This study concluded that dependent men were more likely to develop a number of diseases, including prostate and other cancers.[16]

What would be the practical implications if a holistic perspective gained more research support and was incorporated into the medical view of prostate cancer? First, the promotion of anxiety–producing examinations and tests would cease, at least until we had definite proof of their usefulness. In June 1999 the U.S. Postal Service planned to issue a stamp urging "annual checkups and tests" for cancer of the prostate. the *New England Journal of Medicine* warned against such foolishness, pointing out that the message was "inconsistent with current scientific evidence and thinking within the medical community."[17] Second, we would not subject tens of thousands of men to invasive and potentially harmful surgery and other equally unproven interventions without fully informing them of the uncertainty that shrouds the treatment of prostate cancer.

A holistic approach that places the person at the centre, rather than the blood test or the pathology report, takes into account an individual life history. It encourages people to examine carefully each of the stresses they face, both those in their environment and those generated internally. In this scenario the diagnosis of prostate cancer could serve as a wake-up call rather than simply a threat. In addition to whatever treatment they may choose to receive or not receive, men who are encouraged to respond reflectively, taking into account every aspect of their lives, probably increase their chances of survival.

A transformation appears to have affected Rudy Giuliani, diagnosed with prostate cancer in April 2000, in the midst of his Senate race against Hillary Clinton. The former mayor of New York City has been described as a driven man, "a robo-mayor immune to fatigue, fear, or self-doubt," who "lived and breathed the work ethic."[18] He completely identified with his role, slept only four hours a day and worked most of the other twenty. It was said of him that he could not abide being away from the centre of the action. He had to have a hand in everything, needing to be in control, "barking orders like a general." He had failed to show compassion to suffering individuals and groups and had displayed emotional tightness to an extreme degree. After his diagnosis, he made a remarkable public confession. Referring to his cancer, he said:

It makes you figure out what you're all about and what's really important to you and what should be important to you—you know, where the core of you really exists. And I guess because I've been in public life for so long and politics, I used to think the core of me was in politics. . . . It isn't.

There is something good that comes out of this. A lot of good things come out of it. I think I understand myself a lot better. I think I understand what's important to me better. Maybe I'm not completely there yet. I would be foolish to think that I was in a few weeks. But I think I'm heading in that direction.

In contrast to prostate cancer, another hormone-related cancer of the male genital tract—that of the testicle—has been a success story of medical and surgical oncology. Whereas this rare disease used to be the third leading cause of cancer death among young men, it is no longer even in the top five. The cure rate with early diagnosis is now over 90 per cent. As the remarkable story of the quadruple Tour de France champion, Lance Armstrong, demonstrates, even men with advanced metastatic disease have hope of full recovery with a judicious combination of surgery, radiation or chemotherapy—and determination.

When I was working in palliative care, an oncologist at the British Columbia Cancer Agency asked me to speak with Francis, a thirty-six-year-old with cancer of the testicle—not because he needed palliation, but because he didn't. Although the tumour had spread to his abdomen by the time Francis was diagnosed, with appropriate treatment he still had a better than fifty-fifty chance of a complete cure. The problem was that he was refusing all medical intervention. The oncologist hoped that my counselling skills might help to reverse his patient's negative attitude.

The medical statistics promising cure—or, at least, prolonged life—did not interest Francis. He based his refusal on religious grounds, arguing that since God sent him this disease, it would be impious of him to resist it. He said he was not afraid of treatment—he simply felt it was wrong to even consider it. I tried to approach his obstinate denial of life from every angle that came to mind. Was it some childhood guilt that he felt merited punishment? It was evident that personally Francis was isolated in life, with no family or close ones. Was he depressed? Was this a form of medical suicide?

I asked, non-believer as I was, whether perhaps it was blasphemous in him to claim to know God's will. If God, indeed, had sent him the cancer, could He not have intended it as a challenge for Francis to overcome and learn from? Further, if God was the source of the illness, was He not finally also the source of the medical knowledge that made a cure highly probable?

I asked all these questions, but mostly I just listened to Francis. What I heard was the voice of a very confused and lonely man who was adamant in his refusal to save his life. He stuck firmly to what he felt were unshakeable religious principles, despite the express disagreement about his ideas from the elders of his church. They told him that his interpretation of their denomination's teaching was wayward and unjustified. They offered to support him through treatment and convalescence, all to no avail.

Francis is one of three or four men I have ever seen with cancer of the testicle. Although the incidence of this malignancy is rising, in the United States there are only about six thousand new cases each year, in Canada about one-tenth that number. There have been no studies of the emotional or personal histories of the men who develop it, only of the psychological consequences. There are remarkable similarities between what little I did learn of Francis's life, the published autobiography of Lance Armstrong and the experiences of Roy, a young man I knew well, whom I interviewed for this chapter.

Armstrong first noticed a slight swelling of his testicle in the winter of 1996 and began to feel uncharacteristically short of breath next spring. His nipples felt sore, and he had to drop out of the 1997 Tour de France owing to a cough and low-back pain. "Athletes, especially cyclists, are in the business of denial," Lance Armstrong writes.[19] It wasn't until September, when he coughed blood and his testicle became painfully enlarged, that he finally sought medical attention. By then the cancer had spread to his lungs and brain.

When it comes to cancer of the testicle, it is not only cyclists who are in the business of denial. Thirty-year-old Roy first felt the swelling in his left testicle in mid-2000 but put off going to his family doctor for another eight months. In the meantime, he told no one. "I was a little embarrassed and secondly I was afraid of getting bad news," he says. According to a British study, such reluctance to get help is not untypical with this disease: "Delayed diagnosis is common, but is more often due to delay in seeking medical advice than to delay in the correct diagnosis being made by the physician. . . . The maximum period of delay between symptoms and orchidectomy was three years, with a . . . mean delay of 3.9 months."[20]

It may be that young men are simply loath to accept that there is anything wrong with them, particularly with their sexual organs. But logic would suggest the opposite: if masculinity were the issue, young men would likely run for help as soon as they noticed an abnormality with their testes—just as they do, for example, when they notice their hair thinning owing to familial baldness. Certainly when we look at Roy's life and at the autobiography of Lance Armstrong, we see deeper motives for the denial of their disease.

I have known Roy and his family since he was eight. I was their doctor for twenty years, until I left my practice in 2000. I discovered that Roy had been treated for testicular cancer when I dropped in for a quick visit to my old office a few months ago. By happenstance it was the same afternoon Roy was there for a checkup. By then I had already read Lance Armstrong's book, *It's Not about the Bike: My Journey Back to Life.* The parallels in the lives of Roy and Lance were eerie. Perhaps the similarities in their response to disease were more than coincidental.

Long before his cancer, Armstrong had developed a pattern of emotional repression. One of his close friends described him as "kind of like an iceberg. There's a peak, but there is so much more below the surface."

Armstrong never knew his biological father, whom he contemptuously dismisses as his "DNA donor." His mother, Linda Mooneyham, the daughter of divorced parents, was seventeen and abandoned when she gave birth to Lance, her first son. Linda's father, an alcoholic Vietnam veteran, gave up drinking, to his credit, the day his grandson was born.

Linda was a spirited and independent-minded young woman but, given her circumstances, also a very needy one, hardly an adult. As Lance was to write, "In a way, we grew up together." When Lance was three, Linda remarried. The stepfather, Terry Armstrong, is described by Lance as "a small man with a large mustache and a habit of acting more successful than he really was." He professed Christian principles but, despite them, beat Lance regularly: "The paddle was his preferred method of discipline. If I came home late, out would come the paddle. Whack. If I smarted off, I got the paddle. Whack. It didn't hurt just physically, but also emotionally. So I didn't like Terry Armstrong. I thought he was an angry testosterone geek, and as a result, my early impression of organized religion was that it was for hypocrites."

As the adolescent Lance was to learn, his stepfather also engaged in extramarital affairs. "I could have dealt with Terry Armstrong's paddle. But there was something else I couldn't deal with," writes Lance, referring to his stepfather's infidelities. The marriage broke up.

Roy is also the first-born, the child of an ill-tempered and violent man who used to beat his wife and his son. "I remember one thing that my dad did. He tied my wrists and tied my ankles and put me out in the backyard. I don't remember how long he left me out there, but what really bothered me was the that guy who lived upstairs was looking out the window at me and laughing at me. How the fuck can you do that to a kid? Obviously it bothers me to this day."

"Was your mom around?"

"I think my mom was at work." Roy looked upon his mother as his ally. Very early he took on the role of defending her against her husband's violence.

Lance Armstrong's mother was also unable to protect her son from being beaten. It is inevitable that a child in that situation would have deep hurt around that failure—and anger not only at the abusive stepfather but also at the mother who could not keep him safe. Lance seems unaware of any such feelings—and that is the source, I believe, of his propensity to deny and ignore his pain. "If it was a suffer-fest," Lance writes about his teenage attraction to endurance sports, "I was good at it."

As indicated in the passage quoted above, he had greater difficulty enduring his mother's betrayal by her husband than his own harsh treatment.

The child of an unhappy mother will try to take care of her by suppressing his distress so as not to burden her further. His role is to be self-sufficient and not "needy"—recall my reflexive suppression of a limp after minor knee surgery. When twenty-five-year-old Lance was given his cancer diagnosis, he was quite unable to tell his mother directly. "I wasn't strong enough to break it to my mother that I was sick," he writes. He accepted the offer of a close friend to inform her on his behalf.

Linda rose to the challenge with great strength, love and courage, supporting Lance through the nightmare of a highly uncertain prognosis, the bewildering difficulties of making the appropriate treatment decisions and the travails of brain surgery and chemotherapy. Her son's automatic reflex to protect her was rooted not in their adult realities but in the childhood experiences that had programmed his coping style.

The result of Roy's childhood relationship with his parents, he says, was that "in the past I've always seemed to put other people's happiness before my own. My self-esteem was very low, so I thought socially that if I made others happy, then they would accept me. I'd try to satisfy them, doing what I thought they would want me to do."

"How would you do that?"

"By not being honest with myself or others. Always going along with what they wanted to do, or not being honest with them if they said something that hurt. I would just let that go.

"A few years ago I had a business with two partners. As far as I was concerned, we were all equal, but it seemed like the way they were running the show, it was all them. They were in charge. My opinion didn't matter. Things like that hurt, but I just suppressed it and kept it in and didn't say anything. I didn't know how to deal with it."

The crucial difference, I believe, between Lance Armstrong and Roy on the one hand, and Francis on the other, is that the first two had had enough love in their lives to hold on to the part of themselves that allowed for the development of a fighting spirit. Unlike Francis, they also both received powerful caring and support from family and friends when they were diagnosed.

I strongly suspect that repression plays a role in the onset of testicular malignancy. It would be worthwhile for someone to undertake a study in which men with the disease were carefully interviewed about how they experienced their lives emotionally. One aspect deserving attention would be the patients' level of closeness to and identification with their mothers. There is—I don't believe coincidentally—an uncanny resemblance in looks between Lance's mother, and his wife, Kik. In a photograph of the three of them in Armstrong's riveting memoir, one can hardly tell the two women apart.

One of the lessons Roy spontaneously drew from his experience of cancer was to refuse to orient his behaviour any longer to pleasing others without considering the cost to himself. "Whatever I do now, it is definitely not to please anyone else," he says. "What is going to make me happy? Is this what I want to do? I've tried it the other way in the past, and it didn't work out for me."

Francis was admitted to palliative care, in the end. The cancer eventually spread to his liver, causing a painful distension of that organ. He died quite soon, sooner than we doctors had anticipated.

9

Is There a

"Cancer Personality"?

T WAS LATE AUTUMN OF 1990 when Jimmy married Linda. The wedding took place in the chapel of Vancouver Hospital's palliative care unit, five days before he died of the skin cancer that had invaded his spine. The bride was eight months pregnant. Except for his father, all Jimmy's family had gathered to witness the ceremony and to be with him in his final weeks. A month and a day after I pronounced Jimmy's death, I attended the birth of their daughter, Estelle, just as I had helped deliver Linda's two older children from her first marriage.

Jimmy wasn't much for doctors. Although he and Linda had been together five years, I had met him only that summer when he visited the office with persistent back pain. It turned out to be the sign of spinal metastases from a skin cancer that had been excised from his leg some years before. The original condition, malignant melanoma, is a life-endangering tumour of melanocytes, the pigmented cells in the skin. A deadly disease with a ready tendency to spread to other organs, melanoma often strikes people in the prime of life.

I did not get to know Jimmy very well, but from our first meeting he impressed me as extraordinarily likeable. He was thirty-one years old, polite and friendly, with sandy-coloured light brown hair, blue eyes, a complexion sprinkled with freckles and a broad, Irish, open-faced look about him.

The exposure of fair-skinned individuals to ultraviolet radiation is the major physical risk factor for malignant melanoma. People of Celtic origin appear to be especially vulnerable, particularly if, like Jimmy, they have light-coloured hair, freckles and blue or grey eyes. Dark-skinned ethnic groups are at little risk for skin cancer—in Hawaii, skin cancer is forty-five times less common among non-Caucasians than in Caucasians.[1] Local dermatologists conduct a "sunscreen patrol" on the beaches of Vancouver in the summertime as a public service, warning sunbathers of the danger they are courting. It is unfortunate that repression is not as easily remediable a problem as inadequate sunscreen. Malignant melanoma has been the subject of some of the most persuasive research evidence linking repression and the development of cancer.

Jimmy's condition deteriorated very quickly, and the chemotherapy and radiation made him feel worse. "I've had enough," he finally said. "This is crazy. I'm dying, and I don't need to be dying as sick as I am." Soon after that, his legs became paralyzed, triggering his admission to palliative care. Death followed within a few weeks. Until I left my practice two years ago, Linda and her children remained my patients. When I called her recently, she agreed to be interviewed for this book, as did Donna, Jimmy's older sister.

I asked Linda to describe her late husband's personality. "Jimmy was easygoing, laid-back and relaxed. He loved to be around people. I had to think when you asked me about what kind of stresses there were in his life. He wasn't a very stressed out kind of person. Now, he was a drinker. He had to drink pretty much every day. That's why I wouldn't marry him all those years, because of the drinking. He had beer every day—at least four or more."

"Did it change him at all?"

"Only if he had a lot more than that. . . . Then he became this very big, lovable bear who wanted to tell everybody how much he loved them. When he drank, he just wanted to hug people. Guys, too, like they were his big brothers. He needed to say to a guy, 'You're my buddy,' and then he would cry.

"He wasn't a violent man, he wasn't angry or frustrated. He was sad. He had a lot of sadness in him, and I don't know why.

"There's only one thing I can think of, some secret that he had about his father that he didn't want to tell me. He couldn't talk about it. He did not talk about his emotions. He did not share anything, really."

"What kind of a childhood had he had?"

"He grew up in Halifax. He always said he was a happy kid. His parents stayed together. Both his parents were alcoholics—the father, from what I understand, drank a lot for a long time. I think the mother started when Jimmy was a teenager."

As I found out later from Jimmy's sister, Donna, his senior by two years, their father had been a heavy drinker throughout their childhood. Donna and I had two conversations. "I felt very comfortable with my childhood," she told me at first. "My younger siblings have a different perspective . . . but I believe we had a very good upbringing. Very happy household . . .

"Jimmy was a real little boy, a happy kid. We'd play all the time. We'd go out into the backyard and have water fights—you know, those little spray guns. I just see him as a kid with a real happy face."

"How do you recall your parents?"

"My father was the nicest, friendliest man around. He was a very funny man. He was always joking around with us, play-fighting with us, tickling. He used to mimic, used to talk like Donald Duck. People would come over and say, 'Get your father to talk like a duck.'

"He was a comical person, but you had to listen to him. We'd joke around with him, but when Dad spoke, the ground shook. . . . When he was annoyed or angry, when enough was enough—that was it. If he told us to do something, you did it."

"Why?"

"Because if not, you'd be punished and yelled at."

Donna married and moved to a different town when she was nineteen. Jimmy stayed with his parents until the age of twenty-two. On what was to have been a brief trip to Vancouver, ostensibly to see a friend, he called to tell his parents he would not be back. He did not return, except for a rare visit.

"He just called and said he wasn't coming home. He left a letter in his top drawer, explaining it."

"He escaped."

"He did. And the reason why, I remember him saying to my parents, 'Hey, I couldn't tell you, because I didn't want to hurt you. . .'"

"So Jimmy had the feeling that it would hurt his parents for him to be an independent person."

"All of us were made to feel that way. For our mother, her children were her world. They were her everything. She tried to do the best she could, but she was very attached to us—even to my detriment but especially to Jimmy's. In retrospect, I realize we were far too attached, to an unhealthy degree. I think at some point you have to let your children go. I think emotionally, she didn't let go. I felt obligated, and many times Jimmy did, too. Normally your parents would try to understand and accept your separateness as you got older."

"Jimmy's escape to the West Coast physically doesn't mean that he liberated himself internally."

"Of course he didn't, no. He felt terrible. He felt very, very bad. He did it, but he also had to live with the feelings."

According to Donna, Jimmy found the burden of his parents' emotional pain unbearable even at the end of his life. "Just before the Labour Day weekend, my brother phoned me. He told me what was going on with the melanoma, but he said, 'You know, Donna, I can't phone Mom and Dad, because emotionally I can't handle it. Could you do it for me?' I said sure, I'll do it. So he said, 'Just make sure that they don't call me all upset and crying and everything, because I couldn't take it.'"

I suggested to Donna that perhaps what she had recalled as Jimmy's childhood "real happy face" might not have been a genuine face at all. At least in part, it could have been a coping mechanism Jimmy adopted in reaction to his parents' anxieties and anger. It was a way of avoiding the painful impact of their emotions on himself. Soothing his parents' feelings was accomplished by negating his own.

Donna called me back a few days later. Our conversation had brought to the forefront many memories. She needed to talk.

"After you and I spoke, I just went on about my day. I went to bed at night. About four o'clock in the morning I woke up. It was just incredible how many things came out and just kept going through my mind.

"You had mentioned Linda saying that Jimmy had a lot of sadness in him, maybe to do with his dad. I knew Jimmy really, really well, and yes, there was a lot of sadness. I can go way back to the beginning, remembering when he was little. The only time I can recall my dad doing anything with my brother was a little bit of roughhousing on the carpet in the living room. And I see a bunch of smiles and laughs. But other than that, there was never any participation in Jimmy's life. Never went to the hockey games. Never played with him.

"The crazy thing is that our father always said that he loved us, but he could be so hurtful. I have a brother who is quite heavy, and he'd ridicule him in front of people. He'd say some terrible things to him. And to Jimmy, too.

"I was never angry with my father—I've always covered up for him, maybe knowingly, maybe in an unknowing way. That night, all of a sudden, I got so angry. I started to think of Jimmy and all the things that happened as he was growing up and throughout his life. I kept thinking of all the times my father raised his voice. If he was trying to fix something and he didn't have the right tools, or the screws fell on the floor, or if something didn't happen exactly the way it was supposed to happen, he would scream and yell, and we were scared. We just fled. All of a sudden I remembered his voice and the screaming and the yelling, and I thought, This is not how you should live. This is not what we should have experienced.

"Even at the end . . . My father came out to see Jimmy—they drove from Halifax. Actually, my sister and her husband did all the driving; my father drank all the way. They arrived a couple of weeks before Jimmy had to go into palliative care. My father walked into the apartment and sat there sipping his beer, not wanting even to go into the bedroom to see his son, to see Jim.

"We were trying to cover up. We didn't want Jimmy to realize that his father couldn't face seeing him—was afraid to see what he was going to look like. Finally, Dad built up enough courage and went into the room, and asked, 'Jimmy, can I get you anything? Is there something that you want?'

"My father came out, went to the fridge, and all of a sudden he said, 'How come there's no apple juice here? I don't believe this!' And he started ranting and raving at all of us in the apartment. We were stunned. Got his coat on and stomped off to the store and came back with apple juice for Jimmy.

"Then my father went home, and that was it. He never saw Jimmy in the hospital. He went back to Halifax and never saw him again. And the funny thing is, well . . . you know Linda was pregnant with Estelle and they got married five days before Jimmy died.

"He was semi-comatose that day."

"Yes, he was drowsy. We'd had to increase his pain medication rapidly."

"Well, one of the things I keep remembering is this. . . . After the wedding, he was weak, but he held his hand up and said, 'Look, look, *just like Dad's ring.*' And his wedding band was identical to my father's. It's funny, those were the words that came out of Jimmy's mouth. *Just like Dad's ring.*"

Jimmy's mode of emotional coping has been extensively documented among melanoma patients. An elegant study in 1984 measured the physiological responses to stressful stimuli of three groups: melanoma patients, people with heart disease and a control cohort with no medical illness. Each person was connected to a dermograph, a device that recorded the body's electrical reactions in the skin as the subject looked at a series of slides designed to elicit psychological distress. The slides displayed statements of an insulting, unpleasant or depressing nature, such as "You're ugly," or "You have only yourself to blame." As their physiological responses were being registered, the participants were asked to record their subjective awareness of how calm or disturbed they felt on reading each statement. The researchers thus secured a printout of the actual level of distress experienced by the nervous system of each subject and simultaneously a report of the subjects' conscious perception of emotional stress.

The physiological responses of the three groups were identical, but the melanoma group proved most likely to deny any awareness of being anxious or of being upset by the messages on the slides. "This study found that patients with malignant melanoma displayed coping reactions and tendencies that could be described as indicating 'repressiveness.' These reactions were significantly different from patients with cardiovascular disease, who could be said to manifest the opposite pattern of coping."[2]

The melanoma group was the most repressed among the three groups; the cardiac patients appeared to be the least inhibited. (It is not, as it may seem, that the reactivity of the cardiac patients is healthy. In between repression and hyper-reactiveness is a healthy median.) This study demonstrated that people can experience emotional stresses with measurable physical effects on their systems—while managing to sequester their feelings in a place completely beyond conscious awareness.

It was in relationship to melanoma that the notion of a "Type C" personality was first proposed, a combination of character traits more likely to be found in those who develop cancer than in people who remain free of it. Type A individuals are seen as "angry, tense, fast, aggressive, in control"—and more prone to heart disease. Type B represents the balanced, moderate human being who can feel and express emotion without being driven and without losing himself in uncontrolled emotional outbreaks. Type C personalities have been described as "extremely cooperative, patient, passive, lacking assertiveness and accepting. . . . The Type C individual may resemble Type B, since both may appear easygoing and pleasant, but . . . while the Type B easily expresses anger, fear, sadness and other emotions, the Type C individual, in our view, suppresses or represses 'negative' emotions, particularly anger, while struggling to maintain a strong and happy facade."[3]

Could it be disease itself that changes someone's personality, affecting his coping style in a way that may not reflect how he had functioned in life before the onset of illness? Jimmy's story, related by his wife and sister, illustrates that repression, "niceness" and lack of aggression are lifelong patterns, having their origins in early childhood. As the researchers who studied physiological stress responses in melanoma patients noted, "When people are diagnosed with a disease—whether cancer or cardiovascular—they do not precipitously change their usual ways of coping with stress or suddenly develop new patterns. . . . Under stress, people usually mobilize their existing resources and defences."

How do psychological stresses translate into malignant skin lesions? Hormonal factors likely account for the fact that the number of melanoma tumours is increasing in bodily sites not exposed to sunlight. Researchers have suggested that hormones may be overstimulating the pigment-producing cells.[4]

The Type C personality traits associated with melanoma have been found in studies of many other cancers as well. In 1991 researchers in Melbourne, Australia, investigated whether any personality traits were a risk factor in cancer of the colon or the rectum. Over six hundred people, newly diagnosed, were compared with a matched group of controls. Cancer patients, to a statistically significant degree, were more likely to demonstrate the following traits: "the elements of denial and repression of anger and of other negative emotions . . . the external appearance of a 'nice' or 'good' person, a suppression of reactions which may offend others, and the avoidance of conflict. . . . The risk of colorectal cancer with respect to this model was independent of the previously found risk factors of diet, beer intake, and family history."[5] Self-reported childhood or adult unhappiness was also more common among the bowel cancer cases. We have already noted similar traits among patients with breast cancer, melanoma, prostate cancer, leukemias and lymphomas, and lung cancer.

In 1946 researchers at Johns Hopkins University began a long-term prospective study to establish whether there are psychobiological characteristics in young people that could help predict susceptibility to future disease states. In the course of the subsequent eighteen years, 1,130 white male students enrolled in medical school underwent psychological testing. They were questioned regarding their emotional coping styles and childhood relationships with parents. Biological data—pulse, blood pressure, weight and cholesterol levels—were also recorded, as were habits such as smoking, coffee drinking and alcohol intake. At study's end, nearly all the subjects had graduated and most were doctors, their ages ranging from thirty to over sixty. At this point, their health status was reviewed; the majority were healthy, but in about equal numbers some had developed heart disease, high blood pressure, mental illness, cancer or had committed suicide.

When the researchers conceived of the project, they had not expected to find that cancer would be associated with any pre-existing psychological factors. However, their data showed just such a connection. There were striking similarities between those who had been diagnosed with cancer and the suicide group: "Our results appear to agree with findings that cancer patients 'tend to deny and repress conflictual impulses and emotions to a higher degree than do other people.'"[6]

The researchers found that both for the healthy majority and for each disease category there was a distinctive set of psychological traits. The lowest scores for depression, anxiety and anger had been originally recorded for the medical students who later developed cancer. They had also reported being the most distant from their parents. Of all the groups, the cancer subjects were the least able to express emotion. Does that mean there is a "cancer personality"? The answer is neither a simple yes nor a no.

Melanoma illustrates the futility of simplistic reductions to a single origin. Fair skin alone cannot be the cause of this cancer, since not everyone with fair skin will develop melanoma. Ultraviolet damage to the skin by itself cannot be sufficient, since only a minority of light-complexioned persons who suffer sunburns will end up with skin cancer. Emotional repression by itself also cannot account for all cases of malignant melanoma, since not all people who are emotionally repressed will develop either melanoma or any other cancer. A combination of these three circumstances is potentially lethal.

While we cannot say that any personality type *causes* cancer, certain personality features definitely increase the risk because they are more likely to generate physiological stress. Repression, the inability to say no and a lack of awareness of one's anger make it much more likely that a person will find herself in situations where her emotions are unexpressed, her needs are ignored and her gentleness is exploited. Those situations are stress inducing, whether or not the person is conscious of being stressed. Repeated and multiplied over the years, they have the potential of harming homeostasis and the immune system. It is stress—not personality per se—that undermines a body's physiological balance and immune defences, predisposing to disease or reducing the resistance to it.

Physiological stress, then, is the link between personality traits and disease. Certain traits—otherwise known as coping styles—magnify the risk for illness by increasing the likelihood of chronic stress. Common to them all is a diminished capacity for emotional communication. Emotional experiences are translated into potentially damaging biological events when human beings are prevented from learning how to express their feelings effectively. That learning occurs—or fails to occur—during childhood.

The way people grow up shapes their relationship with their own bodies and psyches. The emotional contexts of childhood interact with inborn temperament to give rise to personality traits. Much of what we call personality is not a fixed set of traits, only coping mechanisms a person acquired in childhood. There is an important distinction between an inherent *characteristic,* rooted in an individual without regard to his environment, and a *response to the environment,* a pattern of behaviours developed to ensure survival.

What we see as indelible traits may be no more than habitual defensive techniques, unconsciously adopted. People often identify with these habituated patterns, believing them to be an indispensable part of the self. They may even harbour self-loathing for certain traits—for example, when a person describes herself as "a control freak." In reality, there is no innate human inclination to be controlling. What there is in a "controlling" personality is deep anxiety. The infant and child who perceives that his needs are unmet may develop an obsessive coping style, anxious about each detail. When such a person fears that he is unable to control events, he experiences great stress. Unconsciously he believes that only by controlling every aspect of his life and environment will he be able to ensure the satisfaction of his needs. As he grows older, others will resent him and he will come to dislike himself for what was originally a desperate response to emotional deprivation. The drive to control is not an innate *trait* but a *coping style*.

Emotional repression is also a coping style rather than a personality trait set in stone. Not one of the many adults interviewed for this book could answer in the affirmative when asked the following: When, as a child, you felt sad, upset or angry, was there anyone you could talk to—even when he or she was the one who had triggered your negative emotions? In a quarter century of clinical practice, including a decade of palliative work, I have never heard anyone with cancer or with any chronic illness or condition say yes to that question. Many children are conditioned in this manner not because of any intended harm or abuse, but because the parents themselves are too threatened by the anxiety, anger or sadness they sense in their child—or are simply too busy or too harassed themselves to pay attention. "My mother or father needed me to be happy" is the simple formula that trained many a child—later a stressed and depressed or physically ill adult—into lifelong patterns of repression.

Jill, a Chicago filmmaker diagnosed with advanced ovarian cancer, admits to being a perfectionist. A friend of hers told me that she had felt concern during the year prior to the diagnosis as she watched Jill endure a stressful experience. "I felt at the time that this is going to be more than psychologically damaging," the friend said.

"About three years ago Jill got into a collaboration on a video. The production company didn't do a great job. It became a horrendous nightmare for her, because her expectations were that she had to come through on a project. Once she's agreed to it, it has to be very high quality. She spent three or five times as much time as she was compensated for. That was, I believe, a big trigger for Jill's body to say, I can't stand this."

My interview with Jill herself was illuminating for its combination of disarming honesty and psychological denial. Jill told revealing stories of stresses in her relationships with her parents and her spouse, without for a moment accepting that these may have contributed to the onset of her illness. She is fifty, highly articulate, with a tendency to go into a labyrinth of details on every topic. I sensed that was her way of keeping anxiety at bay. She appeared uncomfortable with even brief silences in the conversation. At our first meeting, Jill was still wearing a wig, having lost her hair because of chemotherapy.

She had adopted a mothering role in her marriage. When her husband, Chris, suffered an acute but debilitating illness, she cared for him with maternal concern and devotion, calling the doctors, nursing him at nights, ensuring that he was well looked after while she was at work. All this time she was preparing a presentation she was about to give at a national conference and conducted an evening study group for aspiring filmmakers. She led such a group the night before she left for the conference, packing at two in the morning and catching an early flight.

It was shortly after her stint of caring for her husband that she experienced the first symptoms of ovarian cancer. The contrast in caretaking by husband and wife was dramatic. Chris made no medical inquiries on her behalf over several months, seemingly oblivious to her pain and weight loss, despite that fact that she was "living on Advils." "Strangers in elevators would ask me if I was well," she says. As often happens with ovarian cancer, doctors took several months to arrive at the diagnosis.

The first thing Jill said when informed she had ovarian cancer was "'My poor husband and my poor mother.' I am a pillar of strength for them. I felt sorry for them, because they would lose that support."

The gynecological oncologist explained to the couple that the prognosis for survival past five years was poor, given the stage at which Jill's disease had been diagnosed. Chris was in denial. "He didn't seem to have heard that," Jill says. "I needed to talk about what I just been told, but in the car on the way home Chris just kept saying how we're going to fight and beat this. He actually didn't remember what the specialist had said about the prognosis, not even afterwards. It completely bypassed him."

As she faced her surgery, Jill had to deal with her mother's decision to stay with her. "She was not going to come. She's really used to being the centre of attention, and she doesn't like flying. But everyone was saying to her, 'Your daughter is going into hospital, and you're not going to be there?' So in response to that she had to be a mother and really come."

"If that's how you saw it, how did you feel about her coming?"

"At the very beginning I was happy that she wasn't coming. I didn't want her. I knew she was using me to be a good mother, but I've always taken care of my mother since my dad died—he had asked me to."

"My guess is that you've taken care of her since you were born."

"Okay, since I was born. My dad used to say to me, you know, leave her be. He was so very protective, exasperated with her, but he really loved her in some twisted way. He also had a great understanding of her limitations, and at his own expense he accommodated her as much as he could.

"Once my father picked me up at the airport as I came back from a major work trip to Southeast Asia. I was exhausted. My mother was a teacher, and Dad wanted to drive me to her school. 'So you can say hello to your mom—she's waiting there with all her pupils,' he said. I said, 'No Dad, I don't want to go. I'm very tired. I've had an emotionally draining trip. I just want to go and be by myself.' 'Do this for your mom. You know she is really looking forward to this.' He actually drove me there, and she was waiting with all the kids, and he made me put this rice paddy hat on that I'd bought so that I would entertain them. She was doted on like this all her life—and he knew that she needed to be honoured that way. She could show the kids her daughter had been away, and now she was back to see her. I played that role to please my dad, and it happened all the time."

"Wouldn't you encourage your children to assert themselves, not be drawn into taking care of somebody in that sense? Jill, you've got this serious disease, this major operation coming up, and your mother not only comes, she stays with you a whole month."

"And she's very demanding. For a whole month I was catering to her. You know, it's true, I'm very dutiful, I am really very dutiful. I take care of her. I went through it and talked about it with my friends, and a lot of them said not to let her come.

"It went through my head many times, If one of my kids were having surgery, and if they didn't want me to come, I would accept it. However, I would hope that they would feel comfortable that I would be there. With my mother, if I was going to feel guilty and miserable because I didn't provide for her also, that would have been a greater stress for me."

Jill's recollection of her childhood is not that she was a compliant child but that she was rebellious. "I wasn't such a good kid as an adolescent. My father said that he would never wish that I would have a kid like me. I was quite a handful for them. As a teenager, I was considered very difficult. I did well at university, but I just didn't like school. Then I got married—somebody professional. So I turned out good for my parents, after all."

Jill's mother died last year, since our interview. Her daughter felt a need to look after her even in death. The obituary she wrote eulogized her mother for having travelled a long distance to be with her and to nurse her after her surgery for ovarian cancer.

10

The 55 Per Cent

Solution

FOURTEEN YEARS AGO, when she WAS thirty-nine, Martha travelled from Phoenix, Arizona, to the Mayo Clinic in Rochester, Minnesota, for a second opinion. Her bowel specialist had recommended that the entire large intestine be removed as the only way of controlling her Crohn's disease. "If they said I needed surgery, I was ready to accept that," she says, "but I was reluctant."

For more than a decade and a half, Martha suffered episodes of bleeding from the gut, anemia, fevers, fatigue and abdominal pain. The symptoms began shortly after the birth of her third child. "It was a very busy time in my life, with a lot of confusion. Jerry, my husband, was in his last year of dental school in Montana. I was twenty-three with three kids." The children were four, two and the baby was only five months old. The family had no income yet, so Martha was doing babysitting and whatever other work she could get. After Jerry's graduation, the couple moved to Phoenix, where he set up his dental practice.

"I just wasn't feeling well. Third baby, very tired and drained emotionally. I was completely alone in Phoenix. I had never wanted to come here in the first place. I wanted to live in Montana. And the truth is, he had an affair one night—that's what pushed me over the top. I began to have abdominal pains."

A few months later, the couple returned to Montana for Jerry's graduation ceremony. "By then I was hemorrhaging from the bowel.

I was hospitalized immediately because my mother-in-law worked in a medical clinic and she saw I wasn't well. That was when I was diagnosed with Crohn's disease."

Crohn's is one of the two major forms of inflammatory bowel disease, or IBD. Ulcerative colitis is the other. Both are characterized by inflammation of the bowel but in different patterns. In ulcerative colitis, the more common of the two, the inflammation begins in the rectum and spreads upward. The entire colon may become involved. The inflammation is continuous but confines itself to the mucosa, the superficial layer that lines the gut.

In Crohn's disease, the inflammation extends through the entire bowel wall. Most often the ileum, which is the third and final part of the small intestine, and the colon are affected, but Crohn's may appear in any part of the digestive tract, from esophagus to large intestine. Unlike ulcerative colitis, Crohn's will skip areas of the alimentary canal so that normal tissue alternates with diseased segments. IBD may be associated with inflammation in the joints, the eyes and the skin.

The symptoms of IBD depend on the site of involvement. Diarrhea is common in both diseases, along with abdominal pain. Patients may need to defecate many times during the day or even find themselves incontinent. When the colon is affected, there will be bloody stools or, as in Martha's case, frank hemorrhaging. Especially with Crohn's, patients may experience fever and weight loss. There may be other complications, such as fistulas created by inflammation—tunnels from the intestines to other organs such as the skin or, say, the vagina.

IBD is usually a disease of young people. Although it may occur at any age, most commonly onset happens between the years from fifteen to thirty-five.

Martha's symptoms settled quickly in hospital with a course of cortisone. Soon after being discharged she bled again and had to be re-admitted. "I got a blood transfusion, but when it was time for discharge, I hemorrhaged again. That time I went into shock. I was in intensive care. Then I got back out and tried to pull my life together.

"I realized that I was probably not wanting to come back to the marriage and the home. I couldn't figure out why else I kept hemorrhaging whenever it was time for me to leave the hospital. Why didn't I just leave my husband? I think I must have just been incredibly young.

The truth is that when I did come home, he ended up having another affair. I said, 'I'm going. This is it.' I should have left then, but I stayed. "The next three or four years I was a sick puppy. I was tired a lot. My older one, who would then have been five, was having to help with the other two because I just wanted to sleep most of the time."

"What was your husband doing all the while? What was your relationship like?"

"I've always compromised for him. He has been an angry person, so I was intimidated by him. He physically intimidated me. He never hit me, but he yelled and threatened and was very aggressive. He was also drinking a lot. One time he really humbled me in front of the kids, which was not good at all. He stood right in my face and yelled at me.

"I was a silent sufferer, and he is an incredible manipulator. Everything was always turned on me. I was always made to feel insecure. At times I couldn't believe how he could twist things to have it be all my fault."

"Did anyone suggest to you that there might be any connection between your stresses and your disease?"

"No. No medical person ever suggested that. But at the Mayo they had an interesting questionnaire. They asked, 'Has anything significant happened/or is happening in this past year?' I remember reading it and thinking, Oh gee, for the first time somebody's actually caring about what's going on in my life. It was significant for me."

Medical science considers IBD to be "idiopathic," of unknown causation. Heredity plays a role, but not a major one. About 10 to 15 per cent of patients have a family history of IBD. The risk is estimated to be from 2 to 10 per cent if a first-degree relative has been diagnosed.[1] Patients often intuitively feel there is a connection between their IBD and life stresses, as Martha did with her hemorrhaging. In fact, research shows that "most people with inflammatory bowel disease believe that stress is a major contributor to illness."[2]

For Martha, the immediate stressor in the year before her visit to the Mayo had been the departure of her two teenage daughters, who both left home to attend universities in California. She had relied on them for emotional support. Her husband continued to be emotionally abusive, and by then he had exchanged his drinking for a gambling habit. Once her daughters were gone, surgery became unavoidable. She realized later, through counselling, how emotionally underdeveloped and dependent she had been.

Tim, fifty-two, with ulcerative colitis, acknowledges his obsessive need to please. "I spend a lot of time trying to appease and trying to impress others rather than looking inwardly." He has two older brothers. Neither has settled down to a recognized career. One of them got married only recently, in his fifties. His mother has been critical of his siblings, judgment Tim has been anxious to avoid.

"I feel like I'm the perfect son, who got married, has a house with a picket fence and three kids. Maybe in some way I've been trying to please my mom without really knowing it." A 1955 survey of ulcerative colitis patients found that "colitis patients' mothers were controlling and had a propensity to assume the role of martyr."[3] No one sets out consciously to be a martyr to her children or to be controlling. A less judgmental way to put this would be that the child perceived himself to be responsible for his mother's emotional suffering.

Tim is a stickler for detail. "He overorganizes everything," his wife, Nancy, says. "He drives me crazy always asking me, 'When is your timeline for this? Don't forget to do this.'" The 1955 study, which looked at over seven hundred people with ulcerative colitis, concluded that a high proportion of these patients "had obsessive-compulsive character traits, which included neatness, punctuality, and conscientiousness. Along with these character traits, guarding of affectivity [emotional expression], over-intellectualization, rigid attitudes toward morality and standards of behaviour. . . . Similar personality traits have also been used to describe patients with Crohn's."[4]

Tim says he is very critical of others and of himself—one more trait for which he ends up judging himself. "I am a perfectionist, so I don't think I have that natural human sympathy. I'm more cold. In fifteen years I've never missed work, even when I was running to the toilet twelve or fifteen times a day, with bleeding. An employee yesterday took the day off—his dog died the night before. I was like 'What are you saying—he's not here because his dog died? It was just a dog. Why can't he come to work?' Some of the staff said, 'Haven't you ever owned a dog? Are you heartless or what?' I just couldn't relate."

Dr. Douglas Drossman is an internationally known gastroenterologist, and a professor of medicine and psychiatry at the University of North Carolina at Chapel Hill. He is an associate editor of *Gastroenterology,* the official journal of the American Gastroenterology Association. Dr. Drossman has been a leading advocate of seeing intestinal diseases as expressions not only of disturbed physiology but also of stressed lives. He wrote a seminal article on the subject in 1998. "On the basis of clinical reports, on appraisal of the existing research literature, and clinical experience, I believe there is at least indirect evidence that psychosocial factors do affect disease susceptibility and activity. The most likely mechanism for this to occur would be through psychoimmunological pathways."[5]

The inflammation of IBD is the result of disordered immune activity in the gut. Beyond their functions of digestion and absorption, the intestines are also one of the body's major barriers to invasion. Whatever is in the gut is simply passing through and still belongs to the external world. Only after penetrating the bowel lining do substances and organisms enter the body proper. Since this protective function of the gut tissue is critical to well-being, it is generously supplied with its own local immune system, one that works in coordination with the body's general immune defences.

Inflammation is an ingenious process invoked by the body to isolate and destroy hostile organisms or noxious particles. It does so by tissue swelling and the influx of a host of immune cells and antibodies. To facilitate its defensive function, the lining, or mucosa, of the bowel is in a "state of perpetually controlled or orchestrated inflammation."[6] That is its normal state in healthy people.

The powerful destructive forces of the immune apparatus must be minutely regulated and kept in such a balance that they are able to carry out their policing duties without harming the delicate body tissues they are charged with defending. Some substances promote inflammation; others inhibit it. If the balance is upset, disease can result. A diminished capacity by the gut to mount an inflammatory response would invite life-threatening infections. On the other hand, an inability to dampen inflammation exposes the gut tissue to self-injury. The central abnormality in inflammatory bowel disease would appear to be just such an imbalance of what one journal article calls the "pro-inflammatory and anti-inflammatory" molecules in the bowel lining. Emotional influences acting through the nerve and immune pathways of the PNI super-system could tip the balance in favour of inflammation. As Canadian researchers have pointed out, "many, if not all, aspects of gut physiology may be regulated by neuroimmune factors."[7]

The nervous system is deeply influenced by emotions. In turn, the nervous system is intimately involved in the regulation of immune responses and of inflammation. Neuropeptides, protein molecules secreted by nerve cells, serve to promote inflammation or to inhibit it. Such molecules are found in heavy concentration in the intestines, in the areas most vulnerable to IBD. They are implicated both in the regulation of local inflammation and in the body's stress response. For example, a neuropeptide called *substance P* is a powerful stimulator of inflammation because it induces certain immune cells to release inflammatory chemicals such as histamine and prostaglandins, among many others. In the gut, immune cells are closely associated with nerve cells. Chronically stressful emotional patterns could induce inflammatory disease in the gut, through the mediation of the PNI super-system and the activation of pro-inflammatory molecules by stress.

The gut, or intestinal tract, is much more than an organ of digestion. It is a sensory apparatus with a nervous system of its own, intimately connected to the brain's emotional centres. Everyone intuitively understands the meaning of the phrase "gut-wrenching" as a description of emotionally upsetting events. Many of us can recall experiencing the sore tummy of the anxious child. Gut feelings, pleasant or unpleasant, are part of the body's normal response to the world—they help us to interpret what is happening around us and inform us whether we are safe or in danger. Nausea and pain or a warm, comforting feeling in the tummy are sensations that orient us to the meaning of events.

The gut secretes its own neurotransmitters and is influenced by the body's general hormonal system. The gut also forms an important part of the body's barrier against noxious substances and plays a major role in immune defence. Its functioning is inseparable from the psychological processing that each moment gauges and reacts to the stimuli presented to us by the environment. The ability of gut tissue to maintain its integrity is heavily influenced by psychological factors, and its resistance to inflammation and even to malignant change is also vulnerable to emotional stress. A species of New World monkey, the cotton-topped tamarin, develops ulcerative colitis and cancer of the colon when captured and caged.[8] A 1999 Italian study showed that in ulcerative colitis, "long-term perceived stress increases the risk of exacerbation over a period of months to years."[9]

In 1997 Dr. Noel Hershfield, the Calgary gastroenterologist whose timely letter to the editor sparked my own interest in psychoneuroimmunology some years ago, published an article in the *Canadian Journal of Gastroenterology*. He pointed out that in clinical trials of medications for inflammatory bowel disease, there have been instances of placebo response in the range of 60 per cent and that in others comparing narcotics with placebo drugs for pain control, the number of patients who obtained the placebo effect was consistent at 55 per cent of the response. The 55 per cent figure has been seen in trials of anti-depressant drugs as well. It has been called "the 55 per cent rule."

Most people think of placebo as a simple matter of imagination, a case of "mind over matter." Although induced by thought or emotion, the placebo effect is entirely physiological. It is the activation of neurological and chemical processes in the body that serve to reduce symptoms or to promote healing.

Dr. Hershfield proposes that it could be useful to study what is different about the people who improve on placebos. "What kind of people are they? What kind of environment do they live in? Is there something from their past experience that produces their response? What kind of lives do they lead? Are they content with their existences, upbringings, marriages and relationships with society?" These are questions that few doctors ever ask their patients, either those who recover or those who do poorly. When such questions are posed, the answers are uniformly revealing. Dr. Hershfield's article concluded with a sensible suggestion, radical though it may seem in today's medical climate: "Perhaps we should include instruction to our colleagues and fellows in the psychosocial aspects of illness, the psychodynamics of recovery and the biochemistry of healing, and teach them that all ills of humanity cannot be solved by yet another endoscopy, another biopsy and another 'high tech' procedure that only confirms but does not heal."[10]

A friend of mine, Tibor, suffered an episode of ulcerative colitis— the first and only significant episode he would have—during a time when he was experiencing "a frantic feeling of hopelessness, fear and apprehension." In his early twenties, shortly after the death of his father, he was unexpectedly confronted with the responsibility of having to support his mother and care for his younger sister. His mother, who was in poor health, had been dismissed from her job and appeared to have little prospect of finding another. "I didn't know how I might ever have a life of my own," Tibor recalls. He was rushed to hospital with high fever and bleeding from the colon.

"They gave me a steroid. I was in the hospital for three weeks, but as soon as they started the treatment I began to feel better and enjoy the nurses around me. This was before hospital cutbacks when nurses had time for patients. The doctors made all kinds of dire predictions of what can happen in the long term—illness, cancer, whatever. I said, 'Well, I'm not going to have that happen to me.' I read up on the subject and saw that there were suggestions that ulcerative colitis was psychologically induced and stress related. I got a book on relaxation techniques. I'd lie down and follow the instructions—you know, just relax your toes, relax your legs, relax your whole body.

"I wasn't on medication for long, only in the hospital. They were telling me to follow this diet or that. I thought, I'm not going to live my life that way. For whatever it was worth, I decided I was going to take control of this situation. I also decided that I would not let external stresses get to me and consciously did what I could do to minimize stress in my life. In the thirty years since, I have been fortunate to have no more than the occasional minor episode of diarrhea or bleeding. None have required medications or medical care."

This is not to suggest that the cure for IBD is to lie down and relax one's toes. But significant in my friend's experience was his immediate decision to take charge.

As Dr. Hershfield implies, not the latest technology or miracle drug but encouraging the patient's capacity to heal may provide the ultimate answer to inflammatory bowel disease. The 55 per cent solution.

11

It's All in Her Head

ATRICIA'S ANGER SEEMS FRESHLY ROUSED. "I'm
furious at the doctors. I've been condescended to.
I've been patronized. I've been told to my face that
I'm faking. I've been told that I have to stop going
for second opinions. I've been told that I'm not
feeling pain."

The gallbladder of the salesclerk was removed in 1991, when she
was twenty-eight, but she continued to have abdominal pain. "I had
what I called phantom gallbladder attacks. I had more of that you've-
been-pumped-full-of-air pain. It would expand, and then I'd throw up,
and then I'd feel better for a bit. I'd go to emergency. They would ignore me or say, 'You've got no gallbladder, so you can't be having these
symptoms.' Then I started to develop sensitivities to certain foods, and
I had diarrhea more often."

After many doctors' visits and tests Patricia was diagnosed with
irritable bowel syndrome (IBS). Medical terminology calls IBS a *functional* disorder. *Functional* refers to a condition in which the symptoms
are not explainable by any anatomical, pathological or biochemical
abnormality or by infection. Doctors are accustomed to rolling their
eyes when faced with a patient who has functional symptoms, since
functional is medical code for "all in the head." There is truth in that.
The patient's experience is, in part, in her brain—but, as we will see,
not in the pejorative and dismissive sense that the phrase "all in the
head" implies.

Fiona's medical history and her experience of emergency wards are
remarkably similar to Patricia's. In 1989, in her early twenties, she also
had gallbladder surgery, with no resolution of her abdominal distress.

"Ever since then, I've had these pains. It's just a mind-boggling, sharp spasm, a pain that they've done every test in the book for and have come up with nothing. So they've diagnosed this IBS. There are no problems with diarrhea or constipation, just pain. The pain is way up here."

"That's not IBS, strictly speaking," I note.

"That's what I've said all along. The diagnosis was made back when they called it spastic colon, and then it's been called IBS. It was a doctor in Toronto who diagnosed it. I've had the stomach scopes, the barium X-ray, and they've given me all the medications. They've tried me on three or four of the different meds for it. The pills have never done anything for me.

"I've gone months without having any of these attacks, and then there may be days where I'll have them. Sometimes they last two minutes, and other times they are debilitating and last for hours. They are sharp, absolute, spasm-type pains. It takes my breath away—a really intense pain. These days they're pretty bad. I may have an attack that lasts an hour, but it feels like a year.

"When I was in Toronto, they didn't know what was wrong with me. They'd put me in hospital and connect me to a Demerol drip, so every time I had an attack I could medicate myself. I had nurses tell me I was just there for the attention and so that I could get more narcotics—that I was hooked on them. My response was 'Then stop giving it to me. All it does is make me sleep—that's the only way it helps with the pain.' I hate the stuff."

Although abdominal pain is a prominent feature of irritable bowel syndrome, by the current definition of the disorder, pain itself is not sufficient for the diagnosis. A person is considered to have IBS if, in the absence of other pathology, she experiences abdominal pains along with disturbances of bowel function, such as diarrhea or constipation.[1] The symptoms may vary from person to person, or even for the same individual from time to time. Patricia's disturbed bowel habits, for example, do not follow any single pattern.

"It swings between constipation and diarrhea. There's not much in between. I can go days without going to the bathroom, and when I do go, it's diarrhea. Sometimes it's several times a day, and sometimes I could be in the bathroom for three hours at once. The only consistent thing is that there is no consistency. It is sometimes explosive, sometimes not."

Although they are not essential for the diagnosis, there are other symptoms commonly noted. It is not unusual for IBS patients to describe stool that is lumpy or small and pellet-like or, on the other hand, loose and watery. They may find themselves having to strain and feeling they have not completely evacuated their bowels. They frequently describe passing mucus with their stool. A sensation of bloating or abdominal distension is also common.

Irritable bowel syndrome is said to affect up to 17 per cent of the population in the industrialized world and is the most frequent reason for which patients are referred to gastroenterologists. Interestingly, most people with symptoms that would qualify them for the diagnosis do not consult physicians.

The medical profession's reflexive discomfort with uncertainty immensely complicates life for patients like Patricia and Fiona. We expect people to present us with diseases that fit neatly into symptom categories and bear unequivocal pathological findings. As the gastroenterologist Douglas Drossman points out, "Forty years ago, Renee Fox, a medical sociologist, noted that one of the most difficult transitions for medical students is to accept the uncertainty that is intrinsic to medical practice. But the biomedical model creates uncertainty for these common conditions that are not explained by underlying disease."[2] That uncertainty follows from our innate distrust of the patient's story when we cannot match it with the hard data of physical examination techniques or scans, X-rays, blood tests, scopes, biopsies or electrodiagnostic tools. In such cases, the complainant finds her symptoms dismissed by doctors. Worse, she may be accused of drug-seeking behaviour, of being neurotic, manipulative, of "just looking for attention." IBS patients, as well as people with chronic fatigue syndrome and fibromyalgia, often find themselves in that situation.

Magda, a physician herself, knew better than to go the emergency wards with her debilitating abdominal pains. She, too, was diagnosed with irritable bowel syndrome. "Mostly I had pain and distension. Nobody could find anything wrong with me, so we called it IBS. I had a colonoscopy and everything done. There was just nothing else to find. I guess you could call it a diagnosis of exclusion.

"There was hardly a day that I didn't have a bellyache. Sometimes I was lying on the floor of my office, with heating pads, wondering how I would get through the afternoon and how I would drive myself home. It was extremely severe pain and frequent. I had abdominal pain 80 or 90 per cent of the time. There was not a day that, by mid-afternoon, I didn't have abdominal pain—for years! I'm sure I would have been in emergency many times, too, with the severity of my pain—it's just that I stay away from places like that because I know what happens there. I didn't think anything helpful would happen. I didn't go, but not because of the lack of severity."

When not seen as the patient's neurotic imaginings, the pain of IBS—and of undiagnosed abdominal pain in general—has been, until recently, thought to be caused purely by uncoordinated contractions of the intestines. Hence phrases like *spastic colon*. Now it has been confirmed that dysfunction in these disorders does not lie solely in the gut itself. A key issue is the way that the nervous system senses, evaluates and interprets pain.

Several observations have led to this new understanding of abdominal problems. Of particular interest are new findings on electrical and scan studies of the brain. When parts of the intestine are artificially distended, the response pattern in the brains of persons with functional abdominal pain characteristically varies from the brain activity of subjects who have no complaints of pain.[3]

Pain from distension of the colon or other parts of the intestine can also be studied by inserting an endoscope into the bowel and then inflating a balloon attached to the scope. In such studies, the functional patient groups repeatedly exhibit a hypersensitivity to distension. They report that the pain from this procedure is similar to the pain they usually experience. One study compared the effects of balloon inflation in IBS sufferers and controls. "Balloon inflation to 60 ml caused pain in 6 per cent of control subjects and 55 per cent of IBS patients. . . . Estimated gut wall tension at different volumes was similar in the two groups. *However, the incidence of pain in relation to wall tension was increased by nearly ten-fold in the IBS group."*[4]

Parallel observations have been made elsewhere in the digestive tract, from the esophagus to the small intestine. It appears, then, that in functional abdominal pain, physiological messages from the gut are transmitted by the nervous system and received by the brain in an altered fashion. "There is a new area of investigation for patients with these disorders," Dr. Drossman writes. "After decades of studying how IBS patients are distinguished from normals with regard to their gastrointestinal physiology, we are beginning to see differences in brain physiology."

A type of scan known as positron emission tomography, or PET, measures the activity of brain regions by recording variations in blood flow. When study subjects experience distension of their rectums, a PET scan will indicate which part of the brain registers a response. With rectal distension, or even the anticipation of rectal distension, IBS patients activated the prefrontal cortex, an area not activated in normals.[5]

The prefrontal cortex is where the brain stores emotional memories. It interprets present stimuli, whether physical or psychological, in light of past experiences, which can date as far back as infancy. Activation in this part of the brain means that some event of emotional significance is occurring. In people who have experienced chronic stress, the prefrontal cortex and related structures remain in a state of hypervigilance, on the lookout for danger. Prefrontal activation is not a conscious decision by the individual; rather, it is the result of the automatic triggering of nerve pathways programmed long ago.

In another investigation, the electrical amplitudes of brainwaves evoked by sound stimuli were greater in IBS patients than in controls, again indicating a physiological hypervigilance.[6]

What accounts for these altered nervous-system responses? The answer emerges when we look not only at human organs but at human lives. There is a high incidence of abuse in the histories of patients with intestinal diseases and especially in those patients with IBS and other functional disorders.

In a 1990 study of women patients conducted at the gastroenterology clinic of the North Carolina School of Medicine, 44 per cent of the women reported some type of sexual and/or physical abuse. "Those with abuse history had a four-fold greater risk of pelvic pain, two to three times more non-abdominal symptoms (e.g., headaches, backaches, fatigue), as well as more lifetime surgeries."[7] In a more recent investigation at the same centre, fully two-thirds of the women interviewed had experienced abuse of a physical or sexual nature, or both. Again, abused patients were more likely to undergo various surgeries, such as gallbladder operations, hysterectomies, and laparotomies. They also had "more pain, non-gastrointestinal somatic symptoms, bed disability days, psychological distress, and functional disability compared to those without sexual abuse."[8]

It is self-evident that direct physical trauma—a severe brain contusion or the cutting or bruising of a nerve—could physiologically disrupt the nervous system. But how does psychological trauma exert its effect on the perception of pain?

The nervous system of the gut contains about one hundred million nerve cells—we have as many in the small intestine alone as there are in our entire spine![9] These nerves do more than coordinate the digestion and absorption of food and the elimination of waste—they also form part of our sensory apparatus. The gut responds to emotional stimuli by muscle contractions, blood flow changes and the secretion of a multitude of biologically active substances. Such brain-gut integration is essential for survival. Large volumes of blood, for example, may need to be diverted from the intestines to the heart and to the muscles of the limbs at a moment's notice.

In turn, the gut is abundantly supplied with sensory nerves that carry information to the brain. Quite to the contrary of what was believed until recently, nerve fibres ascending from the intestines to the brain greatly outnumber ones descending from brain to gut.[10]

The brain relays to the gut data from sensory organs such as the eyes, the skin or the ears—or more correctly, relayed to the gut is the *interpretation* of such data by the brain's emotional centres. The resulting physiological events in the gut then reinforce that emotional interpretation. The signals sent back to the brain give rise to gut feelings that we can apprehend consciously. If we lose touch with gut feelings, the world becomes less safe.

Obviously, life would not be livable if we felt every micro-event in our bodies. Digestion, breathing, blood flow to organs or limbs and myriad other functions must take place without intruding on consciousness. There has to be a threshold below which the brain does not register sensation, below which stimuli are accepted as unremarkable but above which the brain will be alerted to potential danger from within or without. There needs to be, in other words, a well-calibrated thermostat for pain and other sensations.

When there are too many "gut-wrenching" experiences, the neuro-logical apparatus can become oversensitized. Thus, in the spinal cord the conduction of pain from gut to brain is adjusted as a result of psycho-logical trauma. The nerves involved are set off by weaker stimuli. The greater the trauma, the lower becomes the sensory threshold. A normal amount of gas in the intestinal lumen and a normal level of tension in the intestinal wall will trigger pain in the sensitized person.

At the same time, the prefrontal areas of the cortex will be in a heightened state of vigilance, responding with distress to normal physi-ological processes. Along with increased pain, IBS patients report higher levels of anxiety, arousal and fatigue during rectal distension than do healthy people. During emotional stress, activity of the cortical regions amplifies the perception of distress.

Dr. Lin Chang is associate professor at the UCLA Medical School and co-director of the UCLA/CURE Neuroenteric Disease Program. He has summarized the current understanding of irritable bowel syn-drome this way: "Both external and internal stressors contribute to the development of IBS. External stressors include abuse during childhood and other pathological stresses, which alter stress responsiveness and make a predisposed individual more vulnerable to developing IBS. Later in life, infections, surgery, antibiotics and psychosocial stressors can all contribute to IBS onset and exacerbation."[11]

Stress can definitely induce contractions of the intestines. Women who have been sexually abused, for example, are prone to constipation when the muscles in their pelvic floor are chronically tight, incapable of relaxing with defecation. Alternatively, as people who have been terribly frightened have experienced, stress can set off uncontrollable movements in the colon. That was graphically illustrated in a young doctor-to-be who became an unwitting guinea pig in an experiment: "The investigators produced an elaborate hoax by suggesting to a fourth-year medical student undergoing a voluntary sigmoidoscopic examination that they were seeing a cancer. This led to increased con-tractility or 'spasm' of the bowel, which persisted until the hoax was explained. These type of studies confirmed that stress affects colonic function in normal persons and patients."[12]

What has been discovered about IBS applies to other diseases of the gut. Patricia, in addition to her IBS, suffers heartburn that has seemed to defy medical explanation. She speaks of it with bitterness. "I have this mysterious gastrointestinal problem that has never been diagnosed. I get acid from eating things that are completely bland. I've had to cut out anything with any flavour from my diet.

"I keep having tests, and they keep telling me I'm fine . . . or, I should say, one test did show a tiny bit of upset, but they tell me it's totally out of proportion to what I actually feel. They put that thing up your nose and down into your esophagus, and they measure the amount of acid. There was, they said, a tiny bit of acid, but not enough to cause the degree of pain I'm having.

"I've been on Pantoloc for about three or four years. It's supposed to wipe out acid completely, and I was only supposed to take it for six weeks. I also take Diovol or Gaviscon every day. I still have symptoms of acid, but they can't find anything."

The medical name for the distressing chronic experience of stomach acid flowing upward into the esophagus is gastroesophageal reflux disease (GERD). Researchers in 1992 studied the relationship of reflux symptoms to stress in subjects diagnosed with GERD. While the perception of reflux-associated heartburn by these patients was markedly increased during the stressful stimuli, the objective measures of acid levels were unchanged from one stimulus to another. Stress, in other words, lowered the pain threshold.[13]

An intestinal specialist unfamiliar with the neurophysiology or psychology of pain who looked at Patricia's lower esophagus through an endoscope could, in good conscience, tell her that the acid reflux he observed was inadequate to explain the degree of her pain. And Patricia, in equally good conscience, would be incensed by what she perceived as the callous dismissal of a symptom that is a source of intense daily discomfort in her life.

This is not to say that people with GERD do not experience more frequent reflux than other people. They probably do, and, once more, it is a brain-gut problem. Investigators comparing healthy controls with reflux patients found that the resting pressure of the esophageal sphincter was more frequently low in the GERD subjects. The decreased efficiency of the sphincter muscles permitted more episodes of reflux.[14]

How can the mind and the brain contribute to reflux? It happens by means of the vagus nerve, which is responsible for the tone of the muscles of the lower esophageal sphincter. In turn, the activity of the vagus is influenced by the hypothalamus. The hypothalamus, as we have seen, receives input from the emotional centres in the cortex that are susceptible to stress. Thus, in GERD, a lower pain threshold is combined with excessive relaxation of the sphincter—both phenomena that can be related to stress.

The three women interviewed for this chapter described similar pain experiences, though it is only Patricia whose constellation of symptoms meet the full diagnostic criteria for IBS. Unlike the majority of patients in the North Carolina studies, none of these women suffered sexual or physical abuse either as children or as adults. How, then, can we explain their lowered pain thresholds?

The downward calibration of the nervous system's pain "thermostat" does not require abuse; chronic emotional stress is sufficient to diminish the pain threshold and to induce hypervigilance in the brain. While abuse would be a major source of such stress, there are other potential stresses on the developing child that are subtle, less visible, but harmful nonetheless. Such strains are present in many families, with parents who love their children and would be horrified by any thought of hurting them. Experiences that affect the physiology of pain perception and of intestinal functioning may happen to children who were not abused in any sense of that word and who even felt loved and protected.

The immediate stressors for Magda's severe abdominal pains were related to her job. At the time she was working in a New York hospital. The director of her laboratory had recently resigned, and Magda was not on good terms with his replacement. "The new boss had it in for me from the beginning. In retrospect, I think she was looking for ways to get rid of me from the day she arrived. It was an extremely unpleasant, tense, miserable situation where I loved my work but I hated the environment.

"I worked incredible hours. I was in at seven in the morning. I usually left on time at four, on principle, unless there was some kind of meeting, which happened quite often. I never stopped for lunch. I never took a break. I took work home; I'd work on weekends. I never added it up, but a lot of hours non-stop with tremendous pressure and dirty, dirty politics and a terrible fear—there were no jobs to go to in my field, which was a dying specialty. I never wanted to do general practice, and I didn't want to go back and do another residency.

"Even with all the pain, I appeared at seven on Monday morning and never dropped the ball—ever. I was never sick. I wasn't going to give them a way to get rid of me. They were never going to find anything wrong. I didn't know what I was going to do with my life. I desperately wanted to leave, but I didn't know what I was going to do."

Magda was born in an East European refugee camp after the war. As the daughter of Holocaust survivors from Poland, she became secondarily traumatized by their experience. She has always carried a heavy burden of guilt and responsibility for the sufferings of her parents and for difficulties they continued to face. Her decision to enter the medical field did not arise from her own inclinations. It was motivated by her perception of the needs and expectations of her parents and by her concern to ease their anxieties for her future security.

"If you look at my natural skills, I'm very good at languages, and I'm very good at explaining things. I would never have gone into medicine if I had been free to choose. In fact, I hated a lot about medicine, but I had to deny it to myself.

"I hated much of the course material. I came within a millimetre of failing anatomy. It was an absolute nightmare. I couldn't do calculus. I couldn't do physics. I don't have that kind of mind. I was never good at clinical work. I don't know if I ever heard a diastolic murmur in my life! I just don't have that kind of skill. I don't think I ever felt a spleen—I just pretended. Those were just not things I was good at or inclined to do.

"I thought that being a doctor was what I wanted. My parents never said I should I do it, or that I shouldn't do something else. They just mentioned enough times that it was so good to be able to help other people, and how even the Nazis needed the doctors."

"Yes, I used to hear that too. And the security that you always carry your knowledge with you in a bag."

"That's right, and nobody can take that away. No matter what kind of times, no matter what happens, doctors are always needed. You can be your own boss and how nice that is. My parents brainwashed me from a very young age.

"Then I became a laboratory researcher and I wasn't a 'regular' doctor the way my parents imagined. My mother never really understood what I did and never really was satisfied. What I do is kind of second rate. I don't put the stethoscope on the patient and I don't write prescriptions, and I don't do all those things real doctors do. I just look at specimens and slides. She doesn't say it to my face, but to some extent she is always disappointed."

As she realized that conventional medical treatment had little to offer her, Magda began psychotherapy. Repressed since childhood, her deep anger toward her parents began to emerge. "I was short-circuiting my visceral experience of anger—at my dad because he yelled and screamed and frightened me so much as a child.

"The much bigger problem was my relationship with my mother. I thought it was wonderful and we were best buddies—she was my friend and my supporter and ally and the one who listened to me for hours when I came home from school, and the one that I felt close to and understood by and all the rest. It took many, many sessions to uncover the fact that this was actually a very poor-quality relationship. With all her protection of me, she undermined me. She left me feeling quite inept socially and within myself, and she didn't help me grow up and become my own person. She kept me—with good intentions—very immature.

"Other things too—she told me stories of the Holocaust. Other kids were told fairy tales, and I was told stories of the Holocaust . . . many inappropriate things."

"Do you feel it was inappropriate for you to find out about that?"

"It was inappropriate at age three and four, when she started telling me. And I don't know what age it was, but I cannot remember a time when I didn't hear the accounts of how the whole family nearly got killed because of me when we crossed the border to escape Poland— about how I cried with everybody except with my mother, but I was heavy and she tripped and fell and dropped me in the river, and in order to save me from drowning, they almost all got shot yelling for help. Then she dislocated her shoulder and it's never been right since.

"My parents never said life would have been easier without a child. They wanted a child—they loved me. But I still took on this sense that I was the problem."

Given the trauma her parents had endured and the circumstances surrounding her developing years, Magda's choice to ignore her own inclinations was almost inevitable. That choice also left her perilously vulnerable to stress. Believing herself to be trapped in a job where she felt rejected by her new laboratory chief was a natural trigger for the excruciating abdominal pains she experienced. In this situation, she could no more assert herself than she could have as a child in her family home. The origin of her pain, as she came to realize, was connected with her unconscious repression of anger.

We have noted that gut feelings are an important part of the body's sensory apparatus, helping us to evaluate the environment and assess whether a situation is safe. Gut feelings magnify perceptions that the emotional centres of the brain find important and relay through the hypothalamus. Pain in the gut is one signal the body uses to send messages that are difficult for us to ignore. Thus, *pain is also a mode of perception.* Physiologically, the pain pathways channel information that we have blocked from reaching us by more direct routes. Pain is a powerful secondary mode of perception to alert us when our primary modes have shut down. It provides us with data that we ignore at our peril.

Fiona, whose abdominal pains were ascribed first to a "spastic colon" and finally to IBS, had a childhood less dramatically charged than Magda's. However, there is a strong emotional resonance in her chronic fear that she was not accepted for who she was.

"I honestly believe now that I'm an adult and I know my dad as an adult that he never intentionally judged me for anything I did, but he was always critiquing and evaluating. I said to a girlfriend of mine in Calgary when I was seventeen that I haven't even had a real job yet and I already felt like my resumé didn't measure up to my sister's and brother's. With Dad it always feels like you're building a resumé instead of just doing what you like to do."

"As a child, did you ever tell your parents when you felt bad?" I inquire.

"Physically, yes. Never emotionally. I've never been good about talking about that. I don't know why. I think it's just too personal and private. I'm better at it now. I would never have talked to you five years ago."

At the time of our interview, the immediate stresses in Fiona's life stemmed from her marriage. She had been in the relationship eight years and there were two children. "My husband suffers from depression and panic attacks. He gets these really anxious moments—he's been like that as long as I've known him. He's a great guy and I love him dearly. He's a kind-hearted person, but it has been so exhausting to look after him. I've been his mother. I have three children—a thirty-nine-year-old, a six-year-old and a two-year-old."

"These are problems you are aware of. Is it possible that the pains you get reflect something else you haven't been paying attention to? Rather than seeing the pains as a problem, perhaps they really are gut feelings that are telling you something. When you don't pay attention to emotional signals, your body says, 'Okay, here are some physical signals for you.' If you don't pay attention to them either, you really are in deep trouble."

A week after that conversation, Fiona called me back. Her husband, she revealed, had a serious drug addiction problem that she had been ignoring for a long time. She had suppressed her anxiety and anger, wanting to hold on to a childlike hope that he would quit. In consequence of our interview, she began to rethink her situation.

Patricia, who suffered from irritable bowel syndrome and esophageal reflux, had the most emotionally difficult childhood of the three women introduced in this chapter. She grew up with a perception not only of being unacceptable as she was but of being unwanted in the first place.

"I know I wasn't wanted. I'm not sure when I first realized it, whether as a teenager or as an adult. I've thought about things that my mom has said to me, and I realized the signs were there since I was a child. I didn't recognize them then. I just knew I felt uncomfortable. She always said, 'You know, I don't think you belong in this family. I think they gave us the wrong baby.' And she'd say it with a smile on her face. But, of course, people often pretend to joke when they say something serious."

Irritable bowel patients are more likely than others to have symptoms elsewhere in the body. Susceptibility to pain—migraines, for example—is a problem many IBS patients are prone to, a fact we can readily understand if we grasp the concept of nervous-system sensitization by stressful experience. Heightened perception of pain can be generalized, as Patricia's medical history illustrates. In addition to IBS and esophageal reflux, Patricia suffers from other conditions, including interstitial cystitis and fibromyalgia.

In the North Carolina study that found a majority of women with IBS to have suffered abuse, it was also learned that in only 17 per cent of the abuse cases was the patient's physician aware of the traumatic history. The practical exclusion of people's life histories from the medical approach to illness deprives doctors of powerful healing tools. It also leaves them vulnerable to grasping at the latest pharmacological miracle. A case in point is the sobering example of a recent "wonder drug" for irritable bowel syndrome.

On October 24, 2000, *The Medical Post,* a weekly publication read by many Canadian physicians, carried an enthusiastic headline: "New Drug Relieves IBS Symptoms in Women." The article reported that a new medication, alosetron, "has been proven in clinical trials to be safe and well-tolerated, and to rapidly and significantly relieve pain and bowel function in patients with IBS, particularly in women with diarrhea-prominent IBS." A leading Canadian authority was quoted endorsing the drug and hoping for others like it to follow: "Physicians are going to potentially have therapies for IBS that are useful. . . . IBS patients have a sense of frustration that we really don't understand what is causing the symptoms. Some of the patients don't get a lot of relief."

Another expert, the head of the department of medicine at a Canadian university, echoed that positive assessment of the newly available medication: "It's a very exciting breakthrough. . . . There is nothing else for them out there. None of the other drugs work. This is it."

Four months earlier, *The Medical Letter,* a respected weekly bulletin on medications, had already reported that there was no evidence alosetron offered any advantages over standard treatment. For those patients who did experience improvement with the medication, the benefits disappeared after one week of stopping the drug. *The Medical Letter* also noted that some women taking it had developed ischemic colitis, a potentially catastrophic condition in which bowel tissue is damaged by a lack of oxygen caused by the constriction of blood supply.

In the United States, too, alosetron had been greeted with much fanfare. It was approved by the Food and Drug Administration in February 2000. At the end of November, only a month after the publication of the enthusiastic article in *The Medical Post,* the FDA forced the manufacturer to withdraw the drug. More women had been hospitalized with ischemic colitis, several of whom required surgery. It was reported that in at least one case the patient's entire colon had to be removed. There were also reports of deaths.

If medications are prescribed in a chronic condition like IBS, they usually have to be taken for months or years. It is always risky to commit to a new drug whose long-term safety cannot have been demonstrated by the time it first appears on pharmacy shelves. Doctors and patients do not have to reach for the pharmacopia when the impact of psychological factors on a disease has so abundantly been demonstrated. There is encouraging research evidence that even minimal psychological intervention can be of benefit: "In one controlled study of cognitive-behavioural treatment for patients with irritable bowel syndrome, eight 2-hour group treatment sessions over a 3-month period led to an increase in the number of effective cognitive and behavioural strategies and concurrent reduction in abdominal complaints. Furthermore, improvement continued at 2-year follow-up examinations."[15]

Magda, the New York physician, has dealt with her debilitating abdominal pains by working out her repressed rage through psychotherapy. She has also entered a profession more suited to her inclinations and personality. "Being in pain 80 per cent of the time disappeared a long time ago," she says. "In the past two or three months, there has been even further improvement. Recently I cleaned out the fridge in my office, where I have a bottle of Bentylol [a medication to relieve spasms of the intestines]. I honestly can't remember when I took the last one. It would be quite a few months ago."

Fiona decided to take the warnings of her abdominal pain to heart. She left her husband when it became clear that he was unwilling to give up his drug addiction. With her two children, she has moved to a new town and filed for divorce. She is no longer experiencing pain.

12

I Shall Die

First from the Top

LZHEIMER'S DISEASE IS BECOMING THE baby boomers' nightmare. Affluence and advanced medical care will ensure that the cohort now entering ripe middle age will live longer than any comparable group in history—and will see more of its members slide into dementia than any previous generation. The number of elderly Canadians is predicted to increase by 50 per cent in the next half century. About 100,000 people die of Alzheimer's annually in the United States, where in 1999 there were estimated to be four million people with the disease. That latter statistic is expected to reach fifteen million in 2050, if present trends continue.

Conditions that lead people to be demented—literally, "out of mind"—become more common as we get older. Three per cent of seventy-year-olds suffer from Alzheimer's or some other form of dementia; by age seventy-seven, the figure rises to 13 per cent. The financial costs are enormous, as is the physical and emotional burden on caregivers. And how can those of sound mind imagine the suffering experienced by someone who helplessly witnesses his memory, his intellect, his very self dissolve into infantile chaos? Gradually comes the loss of control over emotional expression, speech and bodily functions until, if the disease runs its natural course, immobility and death follow.

"This is the worst thing that can happen to a thinking person," a person with Alzhemier's said. "You can feel yourself, your whole inside and outside, break down." The patient was talking to David Shenk, author of *The Forgetting,* an illuminating book on the history of Alzheimer's disease.

Shenk also quotes Jonathan Swift. The seventeenth-century Irish writer, satirist and wit was an intellectual giant reduced in his last years to being a mental Lilliputian, his memory failing, his thoughts disordered. "I neither read nor write, nor remember nor converse," Swift lamented in a letter composed during the early phases of his dementia. In another, he said that he could "hardly write 10 lines without blunders, as you will see by the numbers of scratchings and blots before this letter is done. Into the bargain, I have not one rag of memory."

One of the first structures to deteriorate in Alzheimer's is the hippocampus, a centre of grey matter in the temporal lobe of the brain, located on either side next to the ears. The hippocampus is active in memory formation and has an important function in stress regulation. It is well known that chronically high levels of the stress hormone cortisol can shrink the hippocampus.

Could early life experience, emotional repression and lifelong stress predispose to Alzheimer's? Scientific research indicates so, as does a close look at the lives of people with Alzheimer's—whether common folk or the famous, like Swift or the former U.S. president Ronald Reagan. An interesting clue that early relationships may be crucial in the later development of dementia comes from animal experimentation. Rats who receive gentle handling in infancy suffer virtually no loss of hippocampal cells in advanced age.[1] Their capacity to remember remains intact. By comparison, non-handled rats are more likely to suffer shrinkage of the hippocampus and also exhibit greater memory impairment in old age.

In humans, the widely reported Nun Study found that low linguistic ability in early life had a strong association with dementia and premature death in late life. The retrospective research examined the handwritten autobiographies of a group of young postulants (candidate nuns), completed during their first year in the convent. Their mean age at the time of writing was twenty-three. More than six decades later, researchers asked to see the autobiographical statements each had made, and in addition, these now aged nuns were examined for mental health and acuity. As part of the study, each nun was asked and gave permission for an autopsy to be performed after her death. It turned out that those who had expressed a paucity of ideas and had used less vivid language in their youthful memoirs were proportionately more likely to have developed clinical Alzheimer's as they grew older, along with the characteristic pathological findings in the brain.[2]

Richness or poverty of language is determined by many factors, but dominant among them is the quality of early emotional relationships. The author of the world classic *Gulliver's Travels* hardly appears to have been deprived of linguistic capacity. On a closer look, Jonathan Swift's life and writing both manifest a poverty of *felt* emotional experience and of *direct* emotional expression. His phenomenal powers were largely confined to intellectual ideas and to an acerbic wit so dry that his humour often escaped less sophisticated readers. As we saw with Gilda Radner, wit can be a coping style that blocks conscious emotional pain, camouflages anger and provides a means of gaining acceptance by others.

We can infer the intensely negative emotions agitating Swift, particularly his rage toward women, from the passive-aggressive style of his irreverent satire and from some crudely descriptive passages in his narratives. Swift conjures one of the most physically revolting experiences to befall Gulliver when he has him encounter a female breast in Brobdingnag, the land of giants. In this scene Gulliver observes a wet nurse suckling an infant. "I must confess no Object ever disgusted me so much as the sight of her monstrous Breast, which I cannot tell what to compare with. . . . It stood prominent six Foot, and could not be less than sixteen in Circumference. The Nipple was about half the Bigness of my Head, and the Hue both of that and the Dug so varified with Spots, Pimples and Freckles, that nothing could appear more nauseous."

We understand this disturbing account on a deeper level when we learn that Swift suffered a grievous emotional hurt in infancy, one that he later attributed to his nurse. Swift's father, also named Jonathan, died seven months before his first and only son's birth. When only a year old, Jonathan was separated from his mother, Abigaile. He was not to see her for years. In an autobiographical fragment, Swift claims that the nurse abducted him, but to some biographers that sounds like "a comforting fable." More likely he was abandoned, since, after a brief reunion, his mother left him once more.

Gulliver's encounter with that monstrous breast no doubt represents an intrinsic emotional memory. Here we are faced with the infant Jonathan's despair and anger at the sudden absence of his mother, who—in the infant's preverbal perception—was unaccountably replaced by the detestable nurse and her abhorrent dug.

Jonathan was twenty years old before he met his mother again; it was a meeting he initiated. In a manner often seen in the emotionally repressed, he idealized his mother's memory despite that minimal relationship. In the eulogy he wrote for her, he said, "If the way to Heaven be through piety, truth, justice, and charity, she is there."

Swift's long-repressed anger toward his mother would erupt later not only in misogynistic writings but also in his relationships with women. Toward them he would display a "cold, inexpressive anger," or even physical violence. Sexually he was repressed. A recent biographer, Victoria Glendinning, writes, "With women who were closer to him, the permafrost of the emotions was maintained. A thaw cannot be risked. No one must have power over him—the power to melt self-possession, the power to hurt. . . . The only possible emotional outlets are limited, unthreatening ones with powerless and submissive women."[3]

Swift's lifelong abhorrence of intimacy and his underlying fear of emotional contact or vulnerability are the defensive responses of a child deprived of emotional nurturing, a child who had to learn quickly to fend for himself. "There was, it seems, no one adult who particularly cared for Jonathan, or for whom he particularly cared."

In some highly sensitive individuals there may arise an uncanny prescience of deeply hidden processes at work in the body/mind. We have noted this before, with the cellist Jacqueline du Pré and the dancer Joanne who died of ALS. Thirteen years before his death, while still in good health, Swift predicted his dementia. He wrote in *Verses on the Death of Dr. Swift*:

> Poor gentleman, he droops apace,
> You plainly find it in his face:
> That old vertigo in his head,
> Will never leave him, till he's dead:
> Besides, his memory decays,
> He recollects not what he says;
> He cannot call his friends to mind;
> Forgets the place where he last dined. . . .

He expressed the same premonition on a walk with a friend, seeing a decaying tree: "I shall be like that tree; I shall die first at the top."

Swift died at age sixty-seven, in his time a fairly advanced age. His last years were an inexorable descent into dementia. Even toward the end, he was capable of uttering poignant wisdom—if only unconsciously, by rote. Glendinning writes: "One day during the sad last months—it was Sunday, 17 March 1744—sitting in his chair, he put out his hand to snatch at a knife lying on the table. Anne Ridgeway moved it out of his reach. He shrugged his shoulders, and rocked himself, and said, 'I am what I am.' He repeated the words, 'I am what I am. I am what I am.'"

From diagnosis to death, life expectancy in Alzheimer's averages eight years, regardless of the age when the disease first strikes. In rare instances, that may be as early as the sixth decade. Such was the case of Frau Auguste D., a fifty-one-year-old woman admitted to a Frankfurt psychiatric hospital in 1901 with a history of unexplainable behavioural quirks, emotional outbursts and memory lapses. Her course of irreversible mental and physical debility culminated in her death four years later. There was no known diagnosis, but posthumously, Frau D.'s condition came to bear the name of her psychiatrist, the brilliant Alois Alzheimer.

Although Frau D.'s deterioration mimicked senile dementia, which was previously thought to be a normal, if unfortunate, consequence of aging, his patient's relatively young age suggested to Alzheimer that she had a yet-unidentified disease process. The new laboratory techniques of the time made possible a post-mortem examination of Frau D.'s brain, yielding what are now recognized as the hallmarks of the diagnosis: pathological changes in brain tissue specific to this disease. Normal nerve fibres are obliterated, replaced by tangles of strange strands called *fibrils* and by plaques, which David Shenk describes as "crusty brown lumps . . . a hodgepodge of granules and short, crooked threads, as if they were sticky magnets for microscopic trash."[4]

Following on Alzheimer's pioneering work, we now know dementia is not an inexorable part of getting older but always represents disease. Various theories have been floated to explain the cause of Alzheimer's, but so far none of them have been convincing. Some years ago, the finding that the Alzheimer's-affected brain contains higher than normal levels of aluminum prompted many people to discard their aluminum utensils in the hope of warding off the disease. Only later was it recognized that the presence of this metal in the brain was a consequence of the degenerative process, not the cause of it. Even more intriguing, tangles and plaques have been found in the brains of people who, during life, exhibited no signs at all of suffering from Alzheimer's. (Recall that we have seen analogous findings of cancer cells in the breasts of women who had no clinical malignancy, or in the prostates of men dying in healthy old age.) A most telling example came in the recently concluded study of nuns and Alzheimer's disease. "Sister Mary, the gold standard for the Nun Study, was a remarkable woman who had high cognitive test scores before her death at 101 years of age. What is more remarkable is that she maintained this high status despite having abundant neurofibrillary tangles and senile plaques, the classic lesions of Alzheimer's disease."[5]

An international scientific consensus is steadily gaining ground that points to Alzheimer's as one of the diseases on the spectrum of autoimmune conditions, along with multiple sclerosis, asthma, rheumatoid arthritis, ulcerative colitis and many others. Again, these are the diseases in which the body's immune system turns against the self. In autoimmune illness, there is blurring between what is self and *non-self*—foreign matter to be attacked.

"Autoimmune aggression" is how Russian researchers recently characterized the pathological process in Alzheimer's.[6] Canadian physicians have found a higher incidence of other autoimmune illnesses in the families of Alzheimer's patients, suggesting a common predisposition.[7] The inflammation of brain tissue in Alzheimer's—called *inflamm-aging* by a group of Italian scientists—has been successfully slowed by the same anti-inflammatory drugs employed in the treatment of arthritis. Spanish invesigators have found immune-system components, including specialized immune cells and chemicals, in the brain tissue of affected patients.[8] Scientists have identified unique anti-brain antibodies manufactured by the confused immune system. According to Austrian researchers, "There is little doubt that the immune system plays a role in the neurodegenerative process in Alzheimer's disease."[9]

The autoimmune diseases all entail imbalances in the body's physiological stress-regulation system, in particular the hormonal cascade set off by the hypothalamus. This surge of hormones culminates in the release of cortisol and adrenalin by the adrenal glands. Many studies have shown dysregulated physiological stress responses in Alzheimer's, including abnormal production of hypothalamic and pituitary hormones and cortisol. In human beings with Alzheimer's and in animal models of dementia, there is excessive production of cortisol, which is paralleled by the degree of damage to the hippocampus.

Dr. Cai Song is an internationally known researcher at the University of British Columbia and co-author of a recent textbook, *Fundamentals of Psychoneuroimmunology.* "I am convinced that Alzheimer's is an autoimmune disease," says Dr. Song. "It is probably triggered by chronic stress acting on an aging immune system."

The emotional centres in the brain profoundly influence the neurological and hormonal processes of the stress response, as we have seen. The repression of negative emotion—for example, the unconscious grief, anger and loathing Jonathan Swift experienced as a result of early deprivation—is a chronic and significant source of damaging stress. Researchers at the Ohio State University have suggested that in Alzheimer's, as in the other autoimmune conditions, negative emotions provide a major risk factor for the eventual onset of disease.[10]

The world's most famous Alzheimer's sufferer is Ronald Reagan. When Reagan was first diagnosed at the age of eighty-three, six years after the end of his second presidential term, he wrote poignantly in his farewell message to the American people, "I now begin the journey that will lead me into the sunset of my life." It has been a long, sad decline.

Like Swift, Reagan suffered trauma early on. His father, Jack, was an alcoholic. "At four, he could hardly comprehend that his father had been arrested for public drunkenness," avers Edmund Morris in his unorthodox biography, *Dutch: A Memoir of Ronald Reagan.* "Dutch, a dreamy, mild-mannered boy, remained oblivious to the high cost of alcoholism. He did not understand why he and Neil [his brother], on baseball afternoons, were festooned around the neck with sacks of freshly-popped corn and told to 'go sell it down in the amusement park.'"[11]

Morris, a perceptive biographer, was wrong this time—or only partially right. While a young child may not be *cognitively* aware of family disgrace, *emotionally* he is absorbing all the negative psychic vibrations of the stressed family system. An emotional shutdown, a tuning-out of reality, is his brain's most readily available defence. In consequence, the Great Communicator could speak the language of sentiment but not that of genuine emotion. "Really, there are no words" became Reagan's mantra, "his standard cliché to express emotion required of him," writes Morris.

If the shutting-down of emotion occurs early enough, during the critical phases of brain development, the capacity to recognize reality may become permanently impaired. Reagan had lifelong difficulty telling fact from fiction. "He had an inability to distinguish between fact and fancy," a former fiancée recalled—an indication that in the child's mind, and later in the adult's, fancy replaced painful fact. "Reagan's memory was selective," writes the publisher and editor Michael Korda in his own autobiography, *Another Life*, published in 1999:

> He was also known to confuse fiction and reality. There had been the anecdote he had told Medal of Honor winners about the Eighth Air Force bomber pilot who, when his B-17 was mortally hit by flak, ordered the crew to parachute out. Just as the pilot was about to jump from the flaming aircraft himself, he discovered that the ball gunner was trapped in his turret, wounded and unable to get out of the hatch above him, terrified of dying alone. The pilot took off his parachute. . . . and lay down on the floor so that he could put his arm into the turret and hold the dying boy's hand. "Don't sweat it, son," he told the gunner, "we'll go down together," as the plane plunged to the ground.
>
> This brought tears to Reagan's eyes and to the eyes of the Medal of Honor winners. The only problem, as the press soon discovered, was that it had never happened. It was a scene from a movie, which the president had unwittingly transposed to real life.[12]

Similar anecdotes about Reagan abound, as do stories of his poor interpersonal memory. "Dad, it's *me*. Your son. Mike," his first-born child once pleaded with him as Reagan blinked at him uncomprehendingly among a group of fellow students.

The then-future president once described himself as "the calm vacant center of the hurricane." Morris writes that there was always about Ronald Reagan's personality an "immense insularity . . . , the child was already sheathed in a strange calm . . . [a] paralysis of sensibility." The purpose of that defensive and self-induced paralysis is clear. As another woman who rejected the young Reagan's advances said, "I've always known Dutch can't be hurt."

Dutch—Reagan's early nickname from his radio announcer days—
could be hurt. He buried the pain and anger deeply. His resulting emotional repression is nowhere more clearly demonstrated than in Reagan's
description of an incident when, at age eleven, he arrived home to find
his father outdoors, inebriated. "It was Jack lying in the snow, his arms
outstretched, flat on his back. He was drunk, dead to the world. I stood
over him for a minute or two. . . . I felt myself fill with grief for my
father. Seeing his arms spread out as if he were crucified—as indeed he
was—his hair soaked with melting snow, snoring as he breathed, I could
feel no resentment against him."

"I could feel no resentment" reveals the young man's rage at his father.
In psychotherapy one often sees this kind of "confirmation by denial":
the speaker spontaneously reports *not* feeling a certain emotion—usually anger—that he had not been asked about in the first place. This
self-report would be more valid than he knew. While it is true that he
could *feel* no resentment, that was so only because his awareness of feeling
had been impaired long ago. He would be reporting, albeit unwittingly,
that his rage lay beyond the bounds of consciousness. The negative assertion— "I could feel no resentment"—represented an internal conflict
between that rage and the forces of repression.

Reagan's mother was apparently too self-absorbed and overwhelmed
by the stresses of marriage to a philandering and alcoholic husband. She
was unavailable to her children—just as, later, Ronald Reagan would
be unavailable to his children. Often the child's antidote to his anger at
being ignored is to idealize his mother, which is what Reagan likely did.
The depths of his denial become most evident when his mother-sub-
stitute, his devoted second wife and caregiver, Nancy, developed breast
cancer. Their physician, John Hutton, was given the duty of informing
the president. Edmund Morris's notes, from October 1987:

> NR has breast cancer.
>
> John Hutton braced himself to tell RR after the Cab. Meeting
> Oct. 5—"Mr. President, I'm afraid I have rather bad news regarding
> the First Lady's mammogram." Says never before realized the power
> of Dutch's denial. Listened at desk, pen in hand, then softly & stonily:
> "Well, you're the doctors, & I'm confident you'll be able to take care
> of it." End of interview.

John repairs perplexed to residence: "Mrs. Reagan, the President is too stunned to say anything." Stays with her until RR arrives, carrying work. Awkward greetings; no mention of the news. Exit Hutton, even more perplexed.

Such instances do not indicate that the person has no emotions; someone truly lacking attachment could at least pretend to possess some fellow feeling. On the contrary, *the emotions can be too overwhelming to be experienced consciously*—but they are physiologically all the more active. Once more we witness that avoiding the experience of emotion in fact exposes people to greater and longer-lasting physiological stress. Because they are unaware of their own internal states, they are less able to protect themselves from the consequences of stress. Furthermore, the healthy expression of emotion is itself stress-reducing. Stress-induced chronic hormonal and immune changes prepare the physiologic ground for diseases like Alzheimer's.

The emotional poverty, disguised by sentiment, in Reagan's auto-biographical writings in his college years is in dramatic contrast to the rich emotional language of the nuns who survived into old age without Alzheimer's. The correlation between the richly affective accounts written by some young nuns and their later freedom from dementia was remarkable. The ones who wrote with emotional paucity similar to Reagan's ended up with Alzheimer's.

The life histories of all the Alzheimer's patients I looked after during my years of family practice were characterized by repressed emotion. I interviewed several adults who are now taking care of aged parents suffering with Alzheimer's. They all reported early loss or emotional deprivation in their parents' lives. "My mother's father died when she was quite young," one person told me. "I think she was about ten or eleven. The family was living in Vancouver, but her parents sent her up to Gibsons to work in a household that summer. This was back in the thirties.

"My mother was working in Gibsons when her father died. My mom's older sister came up and brought her back to Vancouver. When they arrived home, her mother said to the sister, 'What did you bring her back for?' In front of my mother. It was an astoundingly cruel thing to do."

"A huge amount of tension was always there when I was growing up," a man whose mother also has Alzheimer's recalled. "Things were under the surface. Everything my mother stated was always super-fine, but the body language was 'go away.' She didn't reveal anything. I always felt growing up that I didn't know what was going on."

Other people can observe what the emotionally repressed person holds back from himself. A well-known Hollywood actress who knew the rising movie star Ronald Reagan but remained unmoved by his charms was, nevertheless, "touched by the despair behind his incessant, nervous jocularity," Morris claims.

Morris once asked the president what he had most longed for as a young man. "There was a long silence as he tried to escape the question," the author writes. Reagan finally replied that what he most regretted was not the lack of someone to love him. Rather, he said, "I missed not having someone to love." Morris notes, "I wrote the words down and followed them with a spiral curlicue useful to biographers, meaning, *He feels the opposite of what he says* [italics his]."

13

Self or Non-Self:

The Immune

System Confused

N THE FIRST EDITION OF his classic *Principles and Practice of Medicine,* published in 1892, William Osler suggested that rheumatoid arthritis has "in all probability, a nervous origin." In present-day language, Osler was referring to psychoemotional stress. He noted "the association of the disease with shock, worry, and grief."

No obscure theoretician, William Osler was the best-known medical doctor in the English-speaking world. According to Sherwin B. Nuland, himself a physician and author, Osler "may have been the greatest clinical teacher of any day, and any country." He taught at McGill University in Montreal, Johns Hopkins University Medical School, Baltimore, and at Oxford. In England he was knighted for his contributions to the healing arts. His widely used textbook underwent sixteen editions—the last one in 1947, twenty-eight years after his death.

In 1957 C. E. G. Robinson, a Vancouver internal medicine specialist, cited Osler's words in a brief article in the *Canadian Medical Association Journal.* "I have also been impressed," he wrote, "by the frequency with which chronic or prolonged stress may precede the development of rheumatoid disease. . . . I think that the emotional and psychological aspect of many rheumatoid patients is of first importance."[1]

Dr. Robinson's medical education was still informed by Osler's humane and holistic approach. Now, at the beginning of the twenty-first century, one may search in vain through the mainstream medical texts for any mention of stress in relationship to rheumatoid arthritis or to its fellow autoimmune conditions, all of them characterized by a civil war of the immune system against the body. The omission, tragic for millions of human beings suffering rheumatoid disease of one type or another, is all the more unjustifiable since research has long since established the stress–autoimmune connection and has given us an understanding of many of its potential physiological pathways.

The large and overlapping set of medical conditions called rheumatic diseases include rheumatoid arthritis, scleroderma, ankylosing spondylitis and systemic lupus erythematosus (SLE). In these disorders, and in many others, a disturbed immune system reacts against the body's own tissues, particularly against connective tissues like cartilage, tendon sheaths, the lining of joints and the walls of blood vessels. These illnesses are characterized by various patterns of inflammation that strikes the joints of the limbs or the spine; or surface tissues like skin or the lining of the eyes; or internal organs such as the heart or the lungs or—in the case of SLE—even the brain.

Characteristic of many persons with rheumatoid diseases is a stoicism carried to an extreme degree, a deeply ingrained reticence about seeking help. People often put up silently with agonizing discomfort, or will not voice their complaints loudly enough to be heard, or will resist the idea of taking symptom-relieving medications.

Celia, a woman in her thirties, experienced an episode of arteritis, or generalized inflammation of the arteries, another autoimmune process. Her pain was severe. "For two days I was in so much pain that I was throwing up from the amount of Tylenol and Ibuprofen I was ingesting. My girlfriend said, 'Do you give up yet?' and she took me to emergency."

"'Do you give up yet'—what does that mean?" I wonder.

"I'm stubborn. Whenever I'm sick, I always have this underlying fear that I won't be believed or that I'll be seen as a hypochondriac."

"So here you are, not able to move because of agonizing pain, and you're worried people will think you're a hypochondriac. Let's reverse this situation for a moment. Imagine it was a friend, or your husband, or your child who was suffering such pain. Would you not have acted much more quickly?"

"Yes."

"Why the double standard?"

"I don't know. It goes back a long way, probably. Back to the way I grew up."

The non-complaining stoicism exhibited by rheumatoid patients is a coping style acquired early in life. Celia's anxieties have always been focused on others. Although she herself was abused as a child, her concern was to protect her mother from a series of abusive partners. She was afraid the family would not have enough money or that the outside world would find out about the family violence.

"Mostly I was very worried about my brother becoming a juvenile delinquent or horrible things happening to him."

"What about you?"

"I always felt I somehow could manage it and get through it. I don't want to accept how really upsetting things are. I rationalize it to a point where I can accept it and deal with it. I minimize."

An intensive medical-psychiatric study of people with rheumatoid arthritis conducted for the Maryland Chapter of the Arthritis and Rheumatism Foundation in 1969 concluded that "despite the diversity in the group, the patients' psychological characteristics, vulnerabilities and life conflicts were remarkably similar."[2] One common characteristic was a pseudo–independence, described by the authors as a *compensating hyperindependence.* Celia's rigid belief that she could get through everything by herself was a coping mechanism, a compensation for emotional needs ignored in childhood. A child in her situation survives by pretending to herself, and to the world, that she has no needs she cannot take care of herself. One aspect of that pretence is to reduce the perception of emotional stresses to a child-friendly size, a habit that may then last for a lifetime.

Compensating hyperindependence originating in early role reversal between parent and child also explains Celia's teeth-gritting endurance of physical pain, to the point that a friend had to drag her to the emergency ward with "Do you give up yet?"

In 1969 the British psychiatric researcher John Bowlby published *Attachment,* the first volume of his classic trilogy exploring the influence of parent–child relationships on personality development. "The reversal of roles between child, or adolescent, and parent, unless very temporary, is almost always not only a sign of pathology in the parent," he wrote, *"but a cause of it in the child."*[3] Role reversal with a parent skews the child's relationship with the whole world. It is a potent source of later psychological and physical illness because it predisposes to stress.

Other traits identified in the psychological investigations of people with rheumatoid disease include perfectionism, a fear of one's own angry impulses, denial of hostility and strong feelings of inadequacy. As we have seen, similar traits are said to be associated with the "cancer personality" or with personalities at risk for MS, ALS, or any other chronic condition. None of these traits represent innate features of a person, nor are they irremediably fixed in the individual.

"In the developmental history of these patients a striking finding was the early *effective* loss of one or both parents," according to the Maryland study. The reader will have noticed how often in the personal histories related in this book there was early separation of the parents, abandonment or even the death of a mother or father. Even more universal is *emotional deprivation,* another commonly repeated theme in the research literature. A 1967 Australian study of people with systemic lupus erythematosus reported that: "More patients than controls reported emotional deprivation in childhood associated with a disturbed parent–child relationship within 'unbroken' families."[4]

Like compensatory hyperindependence, the repression of anger is a form of *dissociation,* a psychological process originating in childhood. The young human being unconsciously banishes from awareness feelings or information that, if consciously experienced, would create unsolvable problems. Bowlby calls this phenomenon "defensive exclusion." "The information likely to be defensively excluded is of a kind that, when accepted for processing in the past, has led the person concerned to suffer more or less severely."[5]

In other words, the angry child got into trouble and experienced rejection. The anger and the rejection had to be deflected inside, against the self, in order to preserve the attachment relationship with the parent. That, in turn, leads to the "strong feelings of inadequacy and a poor self-concept" researchers have recognized in people with rheumatoid disease. "Not infrequently anger is redirected away from an attachment figure who aroused it and aimed instead at the self," Bowlby explains. "Inappropriate self-criticism results."[6]

In autoimmune disease, the body's defences turn against the self. In the life of a society—the body politic—such behaviour would be denounced as treason. Within the individual organism, physical mutiny results from an immunologic confusion that perfectly mirrors the unconscious psychological confusion of self and non-self. In this disarray of boundaries, the immune cells attack the body as if the latter were a foreign substance, just as the psychic self is attacked by inward-directed reproaches and anger.

The cross-confusion reflects disruptions of the interconnected body/mind mechanisms within the emotional-nervous-immune-hormonal super-system, which we have called the PNI system.

Emotions precisely parallel and complement the other components of the PNI network: like the immune and nervous systems, emotions safeguard the organism from external threat; like the nervous system and the hormones, they assure the satisfaction of indispensable appetites and needs; and, like all these systems together, they help maintain and repair the internal milieu.

Emotions—fear, anger, love—are as necessary for the organism's survival as nerve impulses, immune cells or hormonal activity. Early on in the process of evolution, primitive responses of attraction or repulsion became essential to the life and reproduction of living creatures. Emotions, and the physical cells and tissues that make them possible, evolved as part and parcel of the apparatus of survival. It is no wonder, then, that the basic molecules that connect all the body systems of homeostasis and defence also participate in emotional reactions. Messenger substances, including endorphins, may be found in the most primitive of creatures who lack even a rudimentary nervous system. It is not that the organs of emotion *interact* with the PNI system—they form an essential part of this system.

In chapter 7 we noted that cytokines, messenger molecules produced by immune cells, can bind to receptors on brain cells to cause changes in body states, mood and behaviour. That emotions induce changes in immune activity is only the other side of the same coin. To illustrate the parallel and complementary protective duties of the emotional system and the immune apparatus, we can compare the role of immune cells with that of an emotion such as, say, anger.

Why do we have anger? In the animal world, anger is not a "negative emotion." An animal experiences anger when some essential need is either threatened or frustrated. Although animals lack conscious knowledge of emotional phenomena, they do feel emotion and experience the physiological changes of Emotion I. And, of course, they manifest the behavioural displays classified as Emotion II. The specific purpose of Emotion I biological changes is to prepare the creature for fight or flight responses. But since flight or fight both demand great expenditures of energy and impose risks of injury or death, the Emotion II displays serve a crucial intermediary function: they often settle the conflict without any of the participants having to get hurt.

A cornered animal turns to face his pursuer with a fierce display of rage. Anger may save his life, either by intimidating the hunter or by enabling the prey to resist successfully. Or anger is aroused in an animal when a stranger of the same species, from outside the family or pack or troop, intrudes on his territory. If the two creatures immediately engaged in physical battle over the disputed territory, one or both would likely become injured. Nature provides a resolution by prompting both of them to mount anger displays: teeth bared, menacing bodily motions, threatening sounds. The more convincing display often wins the day, avoiding harm to either contestant.

For anger to be deployed appropriately, the organism has to distinguish between threat and non-threat. The fundamental differentiation to be made is between self and non-self. If I don't know where my own boundaries begin and end, I cannot know when something potentially dangerous is intruding on them. The necessary distinctions between what is familiar or foreign, and what is benign or potentially harmful, require an accurate appraisal of self and non-self. Anger represents both a *recognition* of the foreign and dangerous and a *response* to it.

The first essential task of the immune system, too, is distinguishing self from non-self. Thus immunity also begins with *recognition*. Recognition is a sensory function, performed in the nervous system by the sensory organs. We may rightly say that the immune system is also a sensory organ. Any failure of the immune system in its responsibility of recognition would expose us to as much danger as we would face if our capacities to see, hear, feel or taste were impaired. Another function of the nervous system is memory. The immune system must also have memory: it needs to recall what in the external world is benign and nourishing, what is neutral and what is potentially toxic.

Under the watchful eyes of the parent, the infant and toddler explore the environment, learning what is edible and what is not, what is comfortable or a source of pain, what is hazardous or safe. The acquired information is stored in the developing brain's memory banks. Immunity is also a matter of learning. Memory is stored by the immune system in cells programmed to recall instantaneously any threat previously encountered. And just as the nervous system must retain its potential for learning throughout the lifetime, so the immune system has the capacity to develop new "memories" by forming clones of immune cells trained specifically to recognize any new threat.

With immune cells found in the bloodstream and in all tissues and spaces of the body, we may think of the immune system as a "floating brain" equipped to detect the non-self. The sensory apparatus—the eyes and ears and taste buds—serving this "floating brain" are receptors on the surfaces of immune cells, configured to know benign from noxious. The self is identified by means of so-called *self-antigens* on the membranes of the body's normal cells, molecules that the immune receptors infallibly recognize. Self-antigens are proteins found on every cell type. Foreign organisms and substances lack such self-markers, making them targets for attack by the immune system. The diversity of self-antigens is just beginning to be discovered. "Chances are that a lot more self-markers will pop up in the future," according to an article in the journal *Science*.[7]

The lymphocytes whose job it is to "remember" foreign antigens are the T-cells that reach maturity in the thymus gland. There are up to a million million of them in human beings. They and their fellow immune corpuscles "must learn to tolerate every tissue, every cell, every protein in the body. They must be able to distinguish the hemoglobin found in blood from the insulin secreted by the pancreas from the vitreous humor contained in the eye from everything else. They must manage to repel innumerable different kinds of invading organisms and yet not attack the body."[8]

It is beyond the scope of this book to discuss the mechanisms by which the various immune cells recognize hostile micro-organisms or other noxious substances and how squadrons of immune cells become programmed to eliminate such invaders. Much has yet to be discovered, and what is already understood involves an extraordinarily complicated sequence of biochemical events, interactions and effects. The point to grasp here is the shared functions of immunity and emotion: first, the "awareness" of self accompanied by an awareness of non-self; second, the appreciation of nourishing inputs and the recognition of threats; finally, the acceptance of life-enhancing influences paralleled by a capacity to limit or eliminate danger.

When our psychological capacity to distinguish the self from non-self is disabled, the impairment is bound to extend to our physiology as well. Repressed anger will lead to disordered immunity. The inability to process and express feelings effectively, and the tendency to serve the needs of others before even considering one's own, are common patterns in people who develop chronic illness. These coping styles represent a blurring of boundaries, a confusion of self and non-self on the psychological level. The same confusion will follow on the level of cells, tissues and body organs. The immune system becomes too confused to know self from other or too disabled to defend against danger.

Ordinarily, immune cells that react against a self-product are immediately killed or inactivated. If immune cells that turn against the self are not destroyed or made harmless, they will attack the body tissues they were meant to guard. Allergic reactions or autoimmune diseases may result. Alternatively, if healthy immune cells are destroyed by radiation, drugs or, say, the HIV virus, the body is left without protection against infections or against the unchecked growth of tumours. Disabling the immune system through chronic emotional stress may have the same effect.

The relationship between self-suppression and immune mutiny was illustrated in a 1965 study of the *healthy* relatives of women suffering from rheumatoid arthritis. Antibodies are normally produced only in response to invasion by microbes or potentially harmful foreign molecules. One of the laboratory hallmarks of rheumatoid arthritis is the finding of an antibody directed against the self by the confused immune system. It is called rheumatoid factor, or RF. Found in over 70 per cent of patients with rheumatoid arthritis, R F may also be present in people without the condition. The purpose of this particular research was to find out whether certain personality characteristics were associated with the presence of the antibody, even in the absence of disease.

Included in the study were thirty-six female adults or adolescents, none of whom had rheumatic disease. Among the subjects, fourteen had the RF antibody. Compared with the women *without* the antibody, the RF-positive group scored significantly higher on psychological scales reflecting the inhibition of anger and concern about the social acceptability of behaviours. They also scored higher on a scale that indicated traits such as "compliance, shyness, conscientiousness, religiosity and moralism."

The presence of the antibody in these subjects suggests that emotional repression had already initiated immune reactivity against the self, although not to the point of clinical disease. One might expect that should additional stressful events occur in the lives of these women, they could further incite the immune mutiny, activate inflammation and trigger frank disease. "Emotional disturbances in conjunction with rheumatoid factor may lead to rheumatoid disease," the researchers concluded.[9] It is also possible to develop rheumatoid arthritis *without* the anti-self antibody RF. As we would expect, in those cases the degree of stress may even have to be greater—precisely as found in another study.[10]

A 1987 review of the literature concluded that "the weight of evidence from a variety of studies strongly suggests a role for psychologic stress in inducing, exacerbating, and effecting the ultimate outcome in rheumatoid arthritis."[11]

Just how specific the effect of stress can be in provoking autoimmune disease is illustrated by the experience of Rachel, a young Jewish woman. Her first episode of rheumatoid arthritis occurred in response to an event that was a re-enactment of childhood emotional trauma.

Rachel had grown up in conflict with her older brother, whom she always perceived to be the favoured sibling. The parents separated, and she felt especially rejected by her father. "I was always the second-class citizen," she says. "It was my brother that he wanted. I still remember walking halfway down the block by myself behind them, my father with his arm around my brother. I remember always having to go into the back seat. I was told by my mother quite a few years ago that I went to Chicago to visit my dad with my brother only because she said, 'You take both kids or you don't take either.' I was never wanted there."

As a child Rachel says she was another "good little girl who never caused any problems," a coping style she continued into adulthood. Two years ago on Rosh Hashanah, the Jewish New Year celebration, she was at her mother's home, preparing dinner for the family. She was in a hurry, since she was to leave in time to avoid meeting her brother, who had decided to join the family at the last moment. "He didn't want to come with me there, so we'd made an agreement that I would go early to my mother's house and help her cook. At 4:00 p.m. I would leave so he and my sister-in-law and niece could spend the rest of Rosh Hashanah with my mother."

"Am I getting this right?" I interjected. "What you're saying is that you would go there and cook and do all the work and then you'd leave so others can have a nice ceremony and a meal together? Why did you accept that arrangement?"

"Because it was Rosh Hashanah and I feel family should be together."

"What happened?"

"When I was at my mother's house, my body went into pain that you wouldn't believe. I was taken to the hospital. The arthritis was in one of my legs, and I couldn't use it at all. I don't usually scream in pain. The whole emergency room heard me, I'm sure. The very next day, I was back at the hospital because it was throughout my whole body. I could not move. Even being wheeled in a wheelchair, I was screaming my head off."

Not only are the onset and flare-ups of rheumatic diseases related to stress but so is their severity. In a study initiated in 1967, fifty young adults newly diagnosed with rheumatoid arthritis were followed over a period of five years. Psychosocial stress factors preceding the onset of the disease were assessed at the beginning. All the patients were examined twice yearly and had annual X-rays of the wrists and hands, the commonest locations of disease activity. At study's end, the subjects were classified according to the degree of tissue damage: in category 1, no swelling on physical examination or X-ray evidence of bone destruction, called erosions; in category 2, soft tissue swelling but no bone erosions; in category 3, bone erosions in the wrists and hands. The results were published in *The American Journal of Medicine*. The researchers observed that the patients who would eventually place in category 3 were, on entering the study, "judged by the interviewers to have a significantly higher frequency of psychosocial stress factors associated with the onset of disease" than those who finished in the other categories.[12]

Most of the interviews I conducted in preparing this book took place in people's homes. Gila, a fifty-one-year-old woman with rheumatoid arthritis, insisted on meeting at the neighbourhood McDonald's outlet. She could serve as the prototype of the "self-sacrificing, conforming, self-conscious, shy, inhibited, perfectionistic" rheumatoid patient described in the psychological literature.

Gila was diagnosed in 1976, during an episode of polymyositis, or generalized muscle inflammation. By the time she sought medical attention, she had lost much of her muscle bulk in her shoulders and hips. Her muscles of respiration were so weakened that she was breathing in a shallow way. She couldn't lift her arms or legs or swallow anything dry. When the specialist saw her, she was hospitalized immediately for a course of intravenous corticosteroid medication. "He said I was a walking corpse. I should not even have been walking around. On my lung-function tests, when I was blowing into the machine, the needle would not move. Not even the slightest movement. But I compensated. You know . . . I didn't realize. When I was walking, I didn't notice that I was swinging, instead of lifting, my leg."

"Why, do you suppose, you didn't notice?"

"I was busy, I guess. I was tired. Because I had two kids, small kids, and I was running around."

"I'm curious why you wanted to meet me at McDonald's."

"At home I'm always self-conscious about how my house looks. It has to be clean and tidy. If somebody comes to my house and notices that there is dust here or there, then . . ."

"You're not talking about tidiness, you're talking about perfection. You can't get away from dust, can you? Dust is part of life. And if you can't accept that, everything has to be perfect. Are you that way with everything?"

"Yeah. Before I had the rheumatoid arthritis actually, I was even more. . . My aunts called me a superwoman. My husband used to go out of town. He had to work in a sawmill for his apprenticeship. I was by myself here with two kids. I worked, and I worked overtime because we just bought a house. Sometimes I worked seven days a week, ten hours a day."

"What did you do?"

"I used to work for the post office. I enjoyed the work, though."

"You liked working ten hours a day, seven days a week?"

"Going to work is almost like going on holiday. I enjoyed the people there. I was friends with the supervisor; nobody gave me a hard time. Although everybody seems to be bored about post-office work around me, I just can't understand why they are bored and complaining. I'm having a good time. So I think that was one of the reasons, too, that I had rheumatoid at first. I think I was abusing myself. I didn't have enough rest. Not enough sleep."

In addition to her job and her housework, Gila also felt she needed to maintain an immaculate garden and backyard. Her home was located between the houses of two retired couples who kept their yards to perfection, and she was concerned that if she neglected her garden their house values would go down. "Yes, impeccable. They would mow every week. So I have to do my lawn every week to keep up." She also was keen for her children to be exposed to opportunities she herself had missed. On weekends she drove them to piano lessons, singing lessons, ballet lessons, folk dancing, sports events.

Gila did all this without any assistance from her husband and, all the while, worked at the post office on the afternoon shift, from 4:30 p.m. until 1:00 a.m. She slept about four hours a night for years. "When I had my rheumatoid arthritis, my physiotherapist told me, 'When you have the pain, you have to stop. You have to rest, because that means your body is telling you that you need to stop.' And so I do that. But the thing is, my housework is not done the way it used to be. Before, I would vacuum every other day, or even twice a day. Now, my husband is the one doing the vacuuming because I can't do it any more. And I'm not happy with the way he vacuums. So sometimes I do it after him, although I don't let him know that. I'm just doing the finishing. My house is not clean or neat and tidy the way it used to be."

Gila was brought up in the Philippines, amid circumstances the reader by now will have guessed. She was the eldest of eight children and the caregiver to all. Her parents criticized her mercilessly. When anything went wrong, she was spanked.

"I had asthma. And every time I got a spanking, the asthma came. And every time I got the asthma, my mom would say, 'Oh, that's God's punishment because you were bad. Because you didn't do your job, because you answered back.' So then I tried to do everything. I was not purposefully being bad. I was doing my best, and I was still being punished when I forgot. And sometimes I just couldn't do it the way she wanted it. She is also a perfectionist."

Gila's husband beat her in the early years of their marriage. Later the abuse lapsed into emotional indifference, but he continues to be morbidly jealous and controlling.

Although some physiotherapists brought up stress issues in their work with Gila, none of the physicians who have treated her for rheumatoid arthritis ever inquired about her personal or emotional life. The wisdom of Sir William Osler has been lost in that vast Bermuda Triangle of modern medical practice.

After she developed her illness, Gila realized she needed to do some psychological work. She understood that her disease, unwelcome as it was, was perhaps trying to teach her something. The medical system was unable to help. At her own request, Gila was referred to a psychiatrist. "He told me that I should not be so upset, that I should treat my husband like he was my oldest son. I didn't go back. I didn't want a third son. I wanted a husband."

In women with rheumatoid arthritis, the immune system has shown increased disturbance during periods of stress, but those who enjoyed better marriage relationships were spared exacerbations of disease activity like inflammation and pain.[13] Another study found that increases in relationship stresses were associated with increases in joint inflammation.[14]

Results like these are not surprising. Recall that stress is a response to a perception of threat. Laboratory studies have demonstrated that many organs and tissues of the body become more vulnerable to inflammation and harm during or after periods perceived as threatening.[15] Stimuli interpreted as potentially dangerous can instantaneously induce dilation of blood vessels, swelling, bleeding, increased susceptibility to

tissue damage and a lowered pain threshold. Such changes can be initiated rapidly in subjects simply by interview techniques that augment
the perception of threat.

There are several potential pathways by which overwhelming
psychological pressures could become manifested as inflammation in
joints, connective tissues and body organs. One of the teachings of the
influential second-century Roman physican Galen was that any part
of the body can affect any other part through neural connections. The
rapid body changes in response to stress are, no doubt, effected through
the instantaneous activity of the nervous system. Discharges originating
in the brain can stimulate faraway nerve endings to release powerful
pro-inflammatory molecules capable of inducing joint damage through
hyperactivity of the immune cells. Some nerve-derived chemicals are
also potent irritating agents for inducing pain. In autoimmune diseases,
elevated levels of some of these substances are found in the fluid of
inflamed joints as well as in the circulation. Such a dramatically quick
mechanism was likely responsible for the acute onset of Rachel's ar-
thritic symptoms as she was labouring over the Rosh Hashanah supper
she was not to attend. The severity of symptoms during that first attack
indicated the severity of her repressed emotional reaction to the situation with her brother.

The *chronic* features of autoimmune disease involve the entire PNI
super-system, particularly the brain-hormone-immune connections.
The hypothesis that stress-induced PNI imbalances are physiologically
responsible for the onset and flare-ups of autoimmune conditions rests
on abundant research evidence.

Elaboration of the many potential mechanisms by which stress acts
through the PNI system to cause autoimmune illness would involve
too much scientific detail for our purposes. Suffice it to say that the
body's stress apparatus, and particularly the production of the key stress
hormone, cortisol, becomes unbalanced through chronic overstimula-
tion. Recall that normal cortisol secretion by the adrenals regulates the
immune system and dampens the inflammatory reactions triggered by
the products of immune cells. In rheumatoid arthritis, there are lower
than normal cortisol responses to stress: we can see why, then, there
would be disordered immune activity and excess inflammation. On the
one hand, the immune system escapes from normal control and attacks

the body to cause inflammation, and on the other, the required anti-inflammatory responses are weakened and ineffective.

It is surely no coincidence that the one medication consistently used in all the autoimmune conditions is the adrenal corticosteroid, cortisol—or, more accurately, its synthetic analogues. Cortisol is the hormone most central to the stress response and the one that studies show to be most disregulated after chronic stress. Autoimmune connective tissue diseases, from SLE and rheumatoid arthritis to scleroderma and ankylosing spondylitis, reflect an exhaustion and disruption of the organism's normal stress-control mechanisms.

Exhaustion is the word that leapt to mind as a former patient of mine with ankylosing spondylitis described his life prior to the onset of his disease, and even after.

Robert is prominent British Columbia labour leader. I interviewed him in his office. A large and affable man in his late forties, Robert speaks with a resonant voice and a hearty humour. When he needs to turn his head to answer the phone or to look at you from a slightly different angle, he swivels his whole trunk. There is virtually no movement in his spine. "Everything's frozen from my neck to my butt," he says.

When he was twenty-five, Robert began experiencing pain in his heels, followed by twelve years of unremitting pain in the joints of his shoulders and collarbone. He went to doctors a few times but soon gave up. "They keep telling you it is this and that, or it is not this or that. They don't give you anything for relief. What else are you going to do about it?" He finally saw a rheumatologist, following five years of pain in his hip and legs.

"I would favour my left leg to the point that I was lying in bed one night and my partner noticed that one leg was smaller than the other—the muscles had shrunk because I didn't use it. Of course, she went into hysterics and made me go to the doctor."

In the twelve years between the onset of his symptoms and his diagnosis, Robert never missed work. In many respects his story was typical. Every trade union official I've ever treated in my practice has been beyond overworked. The demands on their time have been enormous, to say nothing of the inherent stress in the job itself, with the constant conflict and the politics, the long unpredictable hours, meetings, never-ending duties. "Our pension plans in the labour movement are very, very good," says Robert. "The reason we have very good pension plans is that nobody lives to sixty-five to collect their pensions . . . or very few! That's why the pension plan for those of us in the labour movement is so strong. Nobody ever retires."

When his rheumatic disease began, Robert was travelling about 100,000 miles a year by air all over North America. In 1976, which he calls his worst year, he was on the road for a consecutive period of four and a half months. "Never saw home all that time. I was working on a strike in the southern U.S. because I was in an international union that didn't have anybody with the skills needed. I was in Arkansas and Oklahoma and Georgia, working twelve to fourteen hours a day, six days a week." He would sleep during "whatever time was left over."

"What was going on in your personal life?"

"Wife, two kids. Labour movement work always kills marriages. I don't know any of my friends still married to their original wives. There are guys that I started with in 1973—some are dead, but some have had two or three, and one guy has had five marriages! This work just chews them up and spits them out.

"You're never there and never contribute. I feel bad about it now. At the time I was too stupid to feel bad about it. I didn't recognize what I had. I've got a close relationship with my kids now—they're grown up. I don't remember my son very much when he was a teenager and when he was a little child; well, I've got photographs. I didn't even know I had a daughter until she was twenty.

"I don't think I questioned it, because everybody else was doing the same thing. It was just part of the culture. Dead marriages and booze were just common. I was the first one in my peer group to stop drinking."

Robert says he has an addictive personality. "Not just to work. Booze, drugs, women, gambling—the whole nine yards. I haven't had a drink since September 2, 1980, at 7:40 p.m. That was the last time I had a beer. I got tired of waking up on the floor with my tongue stuck to the carpet and feeling like a bag of shit. I've also quit smoking 132 times. Problem is, I've started 133 times. That's the one addiction I haven't been able to break."

What drew Robert to union organizing, and what still keeps him committed to it, is the opportunity to improve people's lives and to work for a more fair, more equitable society. "That's why you never say no. There's always so much more to be done. The list of injustices never gets any shorter. I feel very fortunate to be able to contribute to making this a better world."

Robert has now developed the capacity to say no to excessive demands. Interestingly—and perhaps not coincidentally—he also finds that his ankylosing spondylitis, with the complete fusion of his ribs and his vertebrae, has conferred an unexpected benefit in emotional expression.

"I have an advantage over others in terms of expressing anger. I have a command of the language. I never shout at anybody. I don't have to shout because I can put words right through you just by controlling my breathing. One of the good things about AS is that freezes your ribs, so your ribs are locked in front and back." Robert explains that when people become upset and lose control of their angry responses, they breathe in a very shallow fashion, using the muscles between the ribs to inflate the chest cavity and thus to draw air into the lungs. Because of his AS, he is unable to do that.

"In order to have a stronger voice and more control over the way you speak, you have to breathe with your diaphragm. *You* don't breathe there—you breathe shallowly and your ribs move in and out. *My* gut goes up and down because I have to breathe with my diaphragm. There's much more muscle control in the diaphragm than there is over top of the ribs." It also affords better emotional control and ensures improved oxygen supply to the thinking parts of the brain.

"Before, I had to work at it. As my ribs froze up, I didn't have any choice."

"That's most interesting. Teachers of yogic breathing are always telling us to breathe using the diaphragm. That's the healthy thing to do. Your AS forced you to do that."

"It gives me the power of clarity. You can tell if most people are angry because they shout at you. That's the way, verbally, they can express that they're angry. With my breathing the way it is, I have to speak in shorter sentences, and I can clip words and project my voice rather than yell. Controlling your breathing allows you to control your temper and your anger—and by controlling I mean using it to get to where you want to go."

As Robert spoke, I was struck by the uncanny ability of nature to teach through adult disease lessons that, in a better world, should be learned in childhood and in health.

One study pointed to the intriguing possibility that even the painful inflammation of rheumatoid arthritis could serve a protective function: joint tenderness was significantly related to a *decrease* in stressful events one week later. "The results have important clinical implications," the researchers concluded. "The dynamic interplay between social-conflict events and joint pain describe a homeostatic system in which negative social interaction is regulated through worsening of the disease."[16]

In other words, the flare-up of disease forced patients into avoiding stressful interactions. The body says no.

14

A Fine Balance:

The Biology

of Relationships

PATIENT OF MINE, A CHILD seven years old, was scheduled for cardiac surgery at British Columbia Children's Hospital. She had already undergone two earlier operations for a congenital heart defect. Her parents were well familiar with the routine and wanted one of the rules of the operating room changed. Previously their daughter had been emotionally upset and struggled when she found herself strapped to the stretcher, surrounded by strangers wearing masks, her arm forcibly held as an intravenous catheter was inserted. This time they wished to stay with her until the anaesthetic took effect and she was fully asleep. Although the hospital staff believed that if parents were present the child would be clingy and all the more recalcitrant, they did relent. The anaesthetic procedure was effected without difficulty.

The traditional hospital practice of excluding parents ignored the importance of attachment relationships as regulators of the child's emotions, behaviour and physiology. The child's biological status would be vastly different under the circumstances of parental presence or absence. Her neurochemical output, the electrical activity in her brain's emotional centres, her heart rate, blood pressure and the serum levels of the various hormones related to stress would all vary significantly.

Life is possible only within certain well-defined limits, internal or external. We can no more survive, say, high sugar levels in our bloodstream than we can withstand high levels of radiation emanating from a nuclear explosion. The role of self-regulation, whether emotional or physical, may be likened to that of a thermostat ensuring that the temperature in a home remains constant despite the extremes of weather conditions outside. When the environment becomes too cold, the heating system is switched on. If the air becomes overheated, the air conditioner begins to work. In the animal kingdom, self-regulation is illustrated by the capacity of the warm-blooded creature to exist in a broad range of environments. It can survive more extreme variations of hot and cold without either chilling or overheating than can a cold-blooded species. The latter is restricted to a much narrower range of habitats because it does not have the capacity to self-regulate the internal environment.

Children and infant animals have virtually no capacity for biological self-regulation; their internal biological states—heart rates, hormone levels, nervous system activity—depend completely on their relationships with caregiving grown-ups. Emotions such as love, fear or anger serve the needs of protecting the self while maintaining essential relationships with parents and other caregivers. Psychological stress is whatever threatens the young creature's perception of a safe relationship with the adults, because any disruption in the relationship will cause turbulence in the internal milieu.

Emotional and social relationships remain important biological influences beyond childhood. "Independent self-regulation may not exist even in adulthood," Dr. Myron Hofer, then of the Departments of Psychiatry and Neuroscience at Albert Einstein College of Medicine in New York, wrote in 1984. "Social interactions may continue to play an important role in the everyday regulation of internal biologic systems throughout life."[1] Our biological response to environmental challenge is profoundly influenced by the context and by the set of relationships that connect us with other human beings. As one prominent researcher has expressed it most aptly, "Adaptation does not occur wholly within the individual."[2]

Human beings as a species did not evolve as solitary creatures but as social animals whose survival was contingent on powerful emotional connections with family and tribe. Social and emotional connections are an integral part of our neurological and chemical makeup. We all know this from the daily experience of dramatic physiological shifts in our bodies as we interact with others. "You've burnt the toast again," evokes markedly different bodily responses from us, depending on whether it is shouted in anger or said with a smile. When one considers our evolutionary history and the scientific evidence at hand, it is absurd even to imagine that health and disease could ever be understood in isolation from our psychoemotional networks. "The basic premise is that, like other social animals, human physiologic homeostasis and ultimate health status are influenced not only by the physical environment but also by the social environment."[3]

From such a *biopsychosocial* perspective, individual biology, psychological functioning and interpersonal and social relationships work together, each influencing the other.

Joyce is a forty-four-year-old professor of applied linguistics. Self-imposed stress, she has noticed, is a major factor in the onset of her asthmatic symptoms. "I think every time I've had an episode, it's been when I've taken on more than I can handle. Even though I think I can handle it, somehow my body is saying that I can't.

"I've been a faculty member at the university for a decade. For a number of years I was the only female. Now it has actually changed; I feel my efforts have paid off. There are four women now, which is good, but internally I always had to take on a lot of things. I had to prove myself. They'd never tenured a woman in my department. There was a climate that wasn't that conducive to women's ideas or women professors.

"I was internalizing a lot of 'shoulds.' It was very hard. Not being able to say no was my issue. For me to say no would mean an incredible emptiness, which I was scared about. I've done a lot of things just to fill up the emptiness."

During this past autumn and winter, Joyce's asthma has been particularly troublesome. She has had to use higher than the usual doses of inhaled medications to open the airways and to counteract the inflammation in her lungs. "I realize my illness is making me say no. As part of an exchange I was to be going to Baltimore, and I said, 'No, I can't go.' That's happened other times. I've cancelled things, saying, 'I have an asthma attack, so I can't do it.' I'm still hiding behind something. I'm not willing to just say, 'I won't do it.'"

In asthma, from the Greek root "breathe hard," there is a reversible narrowing of the bronchioles, the small airways in the lungs, because the muscle fibres that encircle them begin to tighten. At the same time, the lining of the bronchioles becomes swollen and inflamed. All the various components of the PNI apparatus are involved in asthma: emotions, nerves, immune cells and hormones. Nervous discharges can narrow the airways in response to many stimuli, including emotions. The immune system is responsible for inflammation of the bronchiolar lining, the other characteristic feature of asthma. Swelling of the airway lining and the accumulation of inflammatory debris in the bronchioles are the final consequences.

It is not inhalation but the outflow of air from the narrowed bronchioles that is impaired in asthma. The asthmatic has difficulty exhaling and feels his chest begin to tighten. The lungs attempt to clear the clogged airways by activating the cough reflex. In acute episodes, the laboured exhalations produce the well-known wheezing noise from the narrowed bronchioles, as from lips puckered for whistling. In milder cases, the only symptom may be an irritating cough. For some people asthma is chronic, while others experience it only intermittently.

Depending on individual predisposition, asthmatic attacks may be set off by everything from allergens to exercise, cold temperatures or medications such as Aspirin, to crying and laughing, viral respiratory infections and emotional arousal. Asthma is one of the few diseases recognized by mainstream medicine to have a significant mind-body component.

Emotions can play a major role in making a person susceptible, no matter what the immediate trigger may be—Aspirin or cold air or anxiety. Chronic emotional stresses sensitize the immune system, so that it becomes overly reactive to any number of triggers.

Another way emotions affect the inflammation in asthma is through hormones. Glucocorticoid hormones—anti-inflammatory steroid hormones, most notably cortisol—are secreted by the adrenal glands on signals from the hypothalamic-pituitary system in the brain. A diminished cortisol response by an impaired HPA axis would promote inflammation. At the University of Trier, Germany, a study found that children known to suffer from atopic dermatitis (eczema, itchy allergic rashes) or from asthma have a diminished production of cortisol in response to stress. "When asked to tell a story or to do mental math, these children show less increase in the glucocorticoid concentrations in their saliva than do healthy peers."[4] In fact, man–made cortisol–like hormones are a crucial part of the treatment for asthma.

Many studies of asthmatic children and adults have documented a strong association between disease severity and emotional states triggered by relationships.[5] Researchers who looked at the interactions between parents and asthmatic children have identified characteristic patterns of insecure attachments. Separation anxiety has been observed in children with asthma to a greater degree, not only in comparison with healthy controls but also when matched with children suffering from cystic fibrosis, a congenital lung disease, more serious by far.[6] The severity of the disease, in other words, was not the cause of the anxiety.

Under test conditions, one study examined the breathing patterns of asthmatic children between two and thirteen years of age, using a comparison group of healthy controls. Each child listened to recordings of his or her mother's voice and that of a stranger. "Regardless of the tone of the voice, asthmatic children showed more abnormal respiratory patterns when listening to their mother's voice than when listening to that of a strange woman. This interesting result suggested a specific emotional effect on breathing that was contrary to what one would have predicted if the child had seen the mother as being reassuring."[7]

In German studies, asthmatic children were more likely than their healthy counterparts to engage in long, escalating, mutually negative interactions with both their mothers and fathers. Their parents tended to exhibit more critical behaviour toward them than the parents of other children.[8] On objective measures, when asthmatic children felt frustrated or criticized, the flow of air from their lungs diminished, indicating airway narrowing. Decreased airflow has also been documented when children with asthma were asked to recall incidents of intense anger or fear.

The stresses that may induce asthma in a child are not necessarily recognized as such by either the patient or the family. Dr. Salvador Minuchin at the Philadelphia Child Guidance Clinic has studied asthma and other childhood illnesses. In his view, highly sensitive children pick up subconscious cues from the environment, particularly about the emotional states of their parents. He has noted that family systems in which children develop disease have four features in common: enmeshment, overprotectiveness (controlling), rigidity and lack of conflict resolution. "A pathologically enmeshed family system is characterized by a high degree of responsiveness and involvement. This can be seen in the interdependence of relationships, intrusions on personal boundaries, poorly differentiated perception of self and of other family members, and weak . . . boundaries."[9]

One of Joyce's recent asthma flare-ups, which lingered several months after the original incident, occurred after a family get-together. The episode, in which she felt attacked by her older brother, brought up emotions of fright and suppressed anger from her childhood.

"When I was young, I operated in fear of the anger that was displayed. I was never hit, but there was a lot of anger around in my family—my father's and my brother's. My mother was complicit in that. She didn't defend me from that anger. The anger wasn't necessarily directed at me, but it was around me. I felt helpless in all of that. Part of my inability to say no has been always that fear of displeasing, of being in difficult situations. Even now, I find it very difficult to deal with problematic situations.

"It was this low level of anger all the time. My father was the righteous one. There would be an expression on his face, a tone in his voice. It was always so irrational, like a child's response to the world. It wasn't like an adult.

"I couldn't take it—I was scared by it. I never felt safe. My father is now eighty-two. He doesn't lash out as much because he's pretty old. My brother is a very angry person; he lashes out all the time and it can be quite devastating.

"Just to say what happened this fall . . . At the end of November is my son's birthday—six years old, and that's a big deal. My parents came up from Seattle, and my brother joined us. We all had dinner together. He just went over the top—critical, angry, directed at me. That happened Friday. Saturday was my son's birthday, and I felt completely upset. I woke up Monday morning and couldn't talk, couldn't walk, couldn't do anything."

A recent Australian study pointed to the importance of positive social relationships in modulating stress. Five hundred and fourteen women who required breast biopsies were interviewed. Slightly fewer than half of the subjects were subsequently diagnosed with cancer, the others with benign tumours. The results "revealed a significant interaction between highly threatening life stressors and social support. *Women experiencing a stressor objectively rated as highly threatening and who were without intimate emotional social support had a ninefold increase in risk of developing breast carcinoma.*"[10]

The investigators found themselves taken by surprise. They write, "Our finding of an interaction between severely threatening life events and the absence of social support was *somewhat unexpected* given the absence of independent effect."

Yet this finding is no more startling than learning that non-swimmers without life jackets are not at risk of drowning—at least, not until they are thrown into deep water. The reader will remember from chapter one that medical students under the stress of exams were shown to have diminished immune system activity, but that the most isolated among them were the most vulnerable. The physiological functioning of human beings is inseparable—even in theory, let alone in practice—from the emotional and social connections that help to sustain us.

A seventeen-year follow-up study of residents of Alameda County, California, looked at the possible links between people's social connectedness or sense of isolation and the onset of cancer. In this prospective study, none of the adults enrolled at the start had cancer. "The risk factor of major interest for women appeared to be social isolation, not only being isolated, but also of *feeling* isolated. . . . Given the effect of emotions on hormonal regulation, it is not unlikely that isolation may have a direct promotional effect on the development of this set of cancers."[11] The researchers grouped cancers of the female breast, ovary and uterus as hormone related.

We do not all mirror one another in how we are physiologically affected by social and interpersonal stressors or other external pressures. What, apart from inborn temperament, accounts for these individual differences?

A key factor is emotional development. Should the child in the first example require a further operation at the age of twenty-five, she will no longer need her mother and father to hold her hand while the anaesthetic is administered. She will have enough self-regulation that neither her neurotransmitter activity nor her stress hormones would go out of balance without her parents' immediate proximity. We cannot take it for granted, however, that with chronological adulthood we automatically attain emotional independence. At any age, our responses to potential stressors are deeply influenced by the degree to which our emotional functioning continues to be dominated by our attachment needs, fears and anxieties.

According to the family systems theory articulated by the late American psychiatrist Dr. Murray Bowen, illness is not a simple biological event in a separate human being. A family systems view recognizes the moment-to-moment interrelatedness of the physiological functioning of individuals. Self-evident in the relationship of mother and fetus, this physiological interrelatedness does not end with birth or even with physical maturation. As we have seen, relationships remain important biological regulators throughout a whole life.

A fundamental concept in family systems theory is *differentiation,* defined as "the ability to be in emotional contact with others yet still autonomous in one's emotional functioning." The poorly differentiated person "lacks an emotional boundary between himself and others and lacks a 'boundary' that prevents his thinking process from being overwhelmed by his emotional feeling process. He automatically absorbs anxiety from others and generates considerable anxiety within himself."[12]

The well-differentiated person can respond from an open acceptance of her own emotions, which are not tailored either to match someone else's expectations or to resist them. She neither suppresses her emotions nor acts them out impulsively. Dr. Michael Kerr, a former colleague of Murray Bowen's, is currently director of the Georgetown University Family Center, Washington, D.C. Dr. Kerr distinguishes between two types of differentiation: *functional differentiation* and *basic differentiation.* The two types may superficially appear to be identical, but from the perspective of health and stress they are worlds apart.

Functional differentiation refers to a person's ability to function *based on his relationships with others.* For instance, it may be that I can do my work well only when other people—my employees, my spouse, my children—can absorb my unresolved anxieties by putting up with my bad temper, unreliable habits, lack of emotional engagement or even abusive behaviour. Were they to reject the roles I assign them, I might fall apart. That would be an example of functional differentiation. On the other hand, if my ability to function is independent of other people's having to do my emotional work for me—that is, if I can remain engaged with others while staying emotionally open to them and to myself—then I would be said to have basic differentiation. The less basic differentiation a person has attained, the more prone he is to experience emotional stress and physical illness.

In a study of stress, adaption and immunity, fourteen hundred military cadets at West Point were followed for four years. They were tested psychologically and had regular blood tests to study their susceptibility to the Epstein–Barr virus, the causative agent for infectious mononucleosis. Those most susceptible to contract the virus or to develop clinical disease had the following in common: they had high ambitions for themselves; they were struggling academically; they had fathers who were high achievers.[13] We can see here the relationship between the stress and the perceived need to live up to parental expectation—that is, between the internal biological milieu and the child's continuing need to gain acceptance.

In another study, married women were matched with an equal number of women who were divorced or separated. In the married group, marital quality and satisfaction were assessed by means of self-reports. Immune system activity was studied in blood samples drawn from each participant. Poorer marital quality was "strongly and positively" related to poorer immune response. In the divorced or separated group, the two psychological factors most closely associated with diminished immune functioning were the time elapsed since the breakup (the more recent the marriage failure, the greater the immune suppression) and the woman's degree of attachment to the former spouse (the greater the emotional attachment, the worse the immune function).[14] Women who were more self-regulated, less emotionally dependent on a relationship that failed to work for them, had stronger immune systems. Greater differentiation means better health.

The less powerful partner in any relationship will absorb a disproportionate amount of the shared anxiety—which is the reason that so many more women than men are treated for, say, anxiety or depression.

(The issue here is not *strength* but *power*: that is, who is serving whose needs?) It is not that these women are more psychologically unbalanced than their husbands, even though the latter may seem to function at higher levels. What is unbalanced is the relationship, so that the women are absorbing their husband's stresses and anxieties while also having to contain their own.

We recall that Nancy, wife of a man with ulcerative colitis, was exasperated at the stress triggered for her by her husband's obsessive and rigid controlling attitudes.* Tim's disease has been in reasonable control over the years. Nancy has effectively absorbed much of his anxiety, but at her own expense. Nancy is now being treated for depression and anxiety and says she is nearing the end of her rope. "It has felt like I have another child," she says, "because he is very high maintenance. I now understand that I have four children I have been responsible for. I'm the parent for both of us. I've repressed my emotional needs for a very long time, without realizing it. It's frightening to think now that I wasn't even aware of that, until I had a mini-breakdown." If Nancy lets go of her one-sided nurturing role in the relationship, Tim may experience a flare-up of his colitis—unless he learns to take more emotional responsibility for himself.

The partner who must suppress more of his or her own needs for the sake of the relationship is more likely to develop physical illness as well—hence the greater incidence, for example, of autoimmune disease and of non-smoking-related cancers among women. "The existence of a mind-body link and a person-person link means that it is possible for *anxiety* in one person to be manifested as a *physical symptom* in another person," Dr. Kerr writes. "As is the case with the emotional dysfunctions, the one prone to develop symptoms is the spouse who adapts most to maintain harmony in the relationship system."[15]

Nature's ultimate goal is to foster the growth of the individual from absolute dependence to independence—or, more exactly, to the interdependence of mature adults living in community. Development is a process of moving from complete external regulation to self-regulation, as far as our genetic programming allows. Well-self-regulated people are the most capable of interacting fruitfully with others in a community

---

* *See chapter 10.*

and of nurturing children who will also grow into self-regulated adults. Anything that interferes with that natural agenda threatens the organism's chances for long-term survival. Almost from the beginning of life we see a tension between the complementary needs for security and for autonomy. Development requires a gradual and age-appropriate shift from security needs toward the drive for autonomy, from attachment to individuation. Neither is ever completely lost, and neither is meant to predominate at the expense of the other.

With an increased capacity for self-regulation in adulthood comes also a heightened need for autonomy—for the freedom to make genuine choices. Whatever undermines autonomy will be experienced as a source of stress. Stress is magnified whenever the power to respond effectively to the social or physical environment is lacking or when the tested animal or human being feels helpless, without meaningful choices—in other words, when autonomy is undermined.

Autonomy, however, needs to be exercised in a way that does not disrupt the social relationships on which survival also depends, whether with emotional intimates or with important others—employers, fellow workers, social authority figures. The less the emotional capacity for self-regulation develops during infancy and childhood, the more the adult depends on relationships to maintain homeostasis. The greater the dependence, the greater the threat when those relationships are lost or become insecure. Thus, *the vulnerability to subjective and physiological stress will be proportionate to the degree of emotional dependence.*

To minimize the stress from threatened relationships, a person may give up some part of his autonomy. However, this is not a formula for health, since the loss of autonomy is itself a cause of stress. The surrender of autonomy raises the stress level, even if on the surface it appears to be necessary for the sake of "security" in a relationship, and even if we subjectively feel relief when we gain "security" in this manner. If I chronically repress my emotional needs in order to make myself "acceptable" to other people, I increase my risks of having to pay the price in the form of illness.

The other way of protecting oneself from the stress of threatened relationships is emotional shutdown. To feel safe, the vulnerable person withdraws from others and closes against intimacy. This coping style may avoid anxiety and block the subjective experience of stress but not the physiology of it. Emotional intimacy is a psychological and biological necessity. Those who build walls against intimacy are not self-regulated, just emotionally frozen. Their stress from having unmet needs will be high.

Social support helps to ameliorate physiological stress. The close links between health and the social environment have been amply demonstrated. In the Alameda County study, those more socially isolated were more susceptible to illness of many types. In three separate studies of aging people, five-year mortality risks were associated directly with social integration: the more socially connected a person was, the lower their risk of death. "Social ties and support," a group of researchers concluded, ". . . remain powerful predictors of morbidity and mortality in their own right, independent of any associations with other risk factors."[16]

For the adult, therefore, biological stress regulation depends on a delicate balance between social and relationship security on the one hand, and genuine autonomy on the other. Whatever upsets that balance, whether or not the individual is consciously aware of it, is a source of stress.

15

The Biology of Loss

ACHEL, WHOSE RHEUMATOID JOINT inflammation first flared on the eve of Rosh Hashanah, is a slight woman, barely five feet tall. Sitting on the sofa in her living room, she is dwarfed by the giant teddy bear propped up beside her. There is something hungry-looking about her, reminiscent of the undernourished and emotionally deprived premature infant she was.

"When I was born, I choked on all the amniotic fluid that had filled my lungs. I spent my first four weeks in a toaster oven of an incubator. Back in 1961 there wasn't the knowledge that infants in incubators still need to be touched. So my first month of life was needles and pokes and prods. My mother didn't come because she had to look after my brother. If my father came . . . I don't know."

The consequences of emotional and tactile deprivation during her first month could have been overcome had Rachel enjoyed nurturing relationships subsequently, but that was not to be. She failed in her appointed life purpose almost from conception. Her mother, who had hoped that the pregnancy would keep the marriage together, was abandoned by her husband even before Rachel's birth. One can imagine the mother's state of mind, being alone and having the sole care of both a toddler—Rachel's brother—and the newborn.

Under such circumstances, having to justify her existence became second nature to Rachel—it is nobody's *first* nature. Her fundamental expectation is that she will be abandoned. "I believe if anybody got to know me, they would leave me for sure," she says. She was astounded when over the last holiday season she received several invitations from people just to visit. That anyone would want her without expecting anything is well nigh impossible for her to fathom.

Since her diagnosis with rheumatoid arthritis, Rachel has entered therapy. As a result, she is much more able than before to know what she feels at any moment. Anger is the emotion she still has the most difficulty recognizing. It is usually roused in her by perceptions of being dismissed or demeaned as, for example, recently when her mother criticized her choice of therapist. "She couldn't understand why I would use a portion of my welfare cheque to pay for therapy rather than go to a psychiatrist funded by the medical plan. So here I have finally found someone I can communicate with, and my mother thinks only about the money part of it." Yet instead of stating calmly that her decisions are her own to make, Rachel argued and pleaded for her mother's understanding. The rancorous exchange induced a week of anorexia, her mode of self-directed rage.

When self-assertion is called for, Rachel swallows her anger and tries to justify herself, to placate or to engage in some interaction designed to persuade the other person to "get it." These efforts are the automatic responses of the vulnerable child who works intensely to bring the parent into alignment with her needs. Her anxiety and fear of abandonment compel her to repress any emotion that may cause her to be rejected.

Rachel's pet rabbit, on the other hand, is acutely sensitive to her owner's emotional states. When Rachel is angry, the rabbit simply refuses be picked up by her. "If I know I'm angry I'll leave her alone. If I am angry but don't know it, she won't let me touch her—she tells me and I'll check in inside, and sure enough I'm angry about something." Although this seems strange to some people, the explanation is straightforward. People and their pets connect via shared brain structures that predate the development of the human frontal cortex with its apparatus of language and rationality. Animals and humans interact from their respective limbic systems, the brain's emotional parts. Unlike people, animals are acutely sensitive to messages from the limbic brain—both their own and that of their owners. In Rachel's unconscious anger the rabbit senses a threat.

How does it come about that a human being would need a rabbit to let her know when she is upset? The simple answer is childhood conditioning. No infant is born with a propensity to repress the expression of emotion—quite the contrary. Anyone who has ever tried to force a baby to swallow foods he disliked or to induce a toddler even to open her mouth when she did not wish to eat can testify to the young human's inherent capacity to resist coercion and to express displeasure. So why do we start swallowing food we do not want or feelings our parents do not want? Not out of any natural inclination but from the need to survive.

Only some aspects of childhood experiences are available to conscious retrieval. Rachel, for example, *recalls* the sense of rejection and humiliation she felt following her father and brother at a distance as the two walked ahead in an embrace. She is also aware of her birth history, although she cannot recall it directly. Yet even without such information, we have infallible testimony about her experience of early childhood: her hopelessness about intimacy; her continued pleas for understanding from her mother, despite nearly forty years of futility; and her reliance on the rabbit as an anger sensor. These behaviours represent an exceedingly accurate memory system, one that was imprinted in her brain in the early stages of her development. That memory system has guided her behaviour all her life and eventually prepared the terrain for the onset of autoimmune disease.

The biology of potential illness arises early in life. The brain's stress-response mechanisms are programmed by experiences beginning in infancy, and so are the implicit, unconscious memories that govern our attitudes and behaviours toward ourselves, others and the world. Cancer, multiple sclerosis, rheumatoid arthritis and the other conditions we examined are not abrupt new developments in adult life, but culminations of lifelong processes. The human interactions and biological imprinting that shaped these processes took place in periods of our life for which we may have no conscious recall.

Emotionally unsatisfying child-parent interaction is a theme running through the one hundred or so detailed interviews I conducted for this book. These patients suffer from a broadly disparate range of illnesses, but the common threads in their stories are early loss or early relationships that were profoundly unfulfilling emotionally. Early childhood emotional deprivation in the histories of adults with serious illness is also verified by an impressive number of investigations reported in the medical and psychological literature.

In an Italian study, women with genital cancers were reported to have felt less close to their parents than healthy controls. They were also less demonstrative emotionally.[1]

A large European study compared 357 cancer patients with 330 controls. The women with cancer were much less likely than controls to recall their childhood homes with positive feelings. As many as 40 per cent of cancer patients had suffered the death of a parent before the age of seventeen—a ratio of parental loss two and a half times as great as had been suffered by the controls.[2]

The thirty-year follow-up of Johns Hopkins medical students was previously quoted. Those graduates whose initial interviews in medical school had revealed lower than normal childhood closeness with their parents were particularly at risk. By midlife they were more likely to commit suicide or develop mental illness, or to suffer from high blood pressure, coronary heart disease or cancer. In a similar study, Harvard undergraduates were interviewed about their perception of parental caring. Thirty-five years later these subjects' health status was reviewed. By midlife only a quarter of the students who had reported highly positive perceptions of parental caring were sick. By comparison, almost 90 per cent of those who regarded their parental emotional nurturing negatively were ill. *"Simple and straightforward ratings of feelings of being loved are significantly related to health status,"* the researchers concluded.[3]

Tactile contact is the newborn's earliest experience of the world. It is how we first receive love. Mammalian mothers invariably provide tactile stimulation to their offspring, for instance, rats by licking their pups, primates by stroking them. Ashley Montague writes in his superb book *Touching: The Human Significance of the Skin,* "The various forms in which the newborn and young receive it is of prime importance for their healthy physical and behavioural development. It appears probable that, for human beings, tactile stimulation is of fundamental significance for the development of healthy emotional or affectional relationships, that 'licking,' in its actual and in its figurative sense, and love are closely connected; in short, that one learns love not by instruction, but by being loved."

From animal experiments, it is known that physical touching induces growth-hormone production, promoting better weight gain and development. These findings also apply to human beings. In a study of premature babies, incubated infants were divided into two groups. All their nutritional and other conditions were identitical, except for one variable: one group was given fifteen minutes of tactile stimulation three times a day over a period of two weeks. "Providing this form of stimulation to these babies resulted in significant acceleration of weight gain, increased head circumference, and improved behavioural indices," compared with the control group.[4] The lack of touching that Rachel experienced impaired her physical development and at the same time gave her the first inkling that she was not desirable or lovable. Later events reinforced those earliest impressions.

Interactions with the world program our physiological and psychological development. Emotional contact is as important as physical contact. The two are quite analogous, as we recognize when we speak of the emotional experience of feeling *touched*. Our sensory organs and brains provide the interface through which relationships shape our evolution from infancy to adulthood. Social-emotional interactions decisively influence the development of the human brain. From the moment of birth, they regulate the tone, activity and development of the psycho-neuroimmunoendocrine (PNI) super-system. Our characteristic modes of handling psychic and physical stress are set in our earliest years.

Neuroscientists at Harvard University studied the cortisol levels of orphans who were raised in the dreadfully neglected child-care institutions established in Romania during the Ceausescu regime. In these facilities the caregiver/child ratio was one to twenty. Except for the rudiments of care, the children were seldom physically picked up or touched. They displayed the self-hugging motions and depressed demeanour typical of abandoned young, human or primate. On saliva tests, their cortisol levels were abnormal, indicating that their hypothalamic-pituitary-adrenal axes were already impaired.[5] As we have seen, disruptions of the HPA axis have been noted in autoimmune disease, cancer and other conditions.

It is intuitively easy to understand why abuse, trauma or extreme neglect in childhood would have negative consequences. But why do many people develop stress-related illness *without* having been abused or traumatized? These persons suffer not because something negative was inflicted on them but because something positive was withheld. As Dr. Myron Hofer, director of the Division of Developmental Psychobiology at Columbia University, wrote in a special edition of the journal *Psychosomatic Medicine* in 1996, "The paradox remains, how could the *absence* of something or somebody create such disturbances. . . . *There must be a biology of loss, and we must find it.*"[6]

How the absence of something or someone creates physiological disturbances becomes clearer if we recall our discussion of stress. All stressors represent the absence, threatened or real, of essential features in the environment, features that the organism perceives as necessary for survival. In "What Is Stress," S. Levine and H. Ursin write that, "Stress stimuli . . . indicate that something is missing or about to disappear and that this something is highly relevant and desirable to the organism."[7]

For any young warm-blooded creature, life is impossible without the parent. The young human depends on adults much longer than the offspring of any other species, for reasons that go well beyond immediate physical needs. Parental caregivers are more than providers of food, shelter, lifeskills information, and protection against predators. As the sad example of the Romanian orphans showed, parents are also the biological regulators of the child's immature physiological and emotional systems. Parental love is not simply a warm and pleasant emotional experience, it is a biological condition essential for healthy physiological and psychological development. Parental love and attention drive the optimal maturation of the circuitry of the brain, of the PNI system and of the HPA axis.

The brain of the human newborn is smaller and less mature, in relation to the adult brain, than that of any other mammal. A horse, by comparison, can run on the first day of life—an activity for which we lack the required nerve circuitry, visual-spatial skills and muscle coordination for another year and a half or more. The straightforward anatomical reason for entering the world so neurologically challenged is the size of our head. Already at birth, the head of the human child is the biggest diameter of the body. It is the part most likely to become stuck in the birth canal. At the same time as the human head grew to accommodate the increasingly complex intellectual and manual-control capacities of the brain, the human pelvis narrowed to permit more balanced two-legged locomotion. One cannot walk two-legged with the pelvis of a horse. Thus, increase in head size co-evolved with the narrowed pelvis; were our brains much larger at the end of gestation, no one would ever be born.

Three-quarters of brain growth and almost 90 per cent of brain development take place following birth, mostly in the first three years of life. Immediately after birth, the human brain, alone among mammalian brains, continues to grow at the same rate outside the uterus as it did inside. In the first months and beyond, there is an astoundingly rapid and complex development of nerve connections, or synapses. We form millions of new synapses a second during some periods.

The unfolding of any developmental process depends not only on inherited genetic potential but also on environmental conditions. The finest and hardiest strain of wheat will fail to grow in barren and dry soil. Decades of neuroscientific research have established that an indispensable requirement of human brain development is nurturing emotional interactions with the parent. Emotional interactions stimulate or inhibit the growth of nerve cells and circuits by complicated processes that involve the release of natural chemicals. To give a somewhat simplified example, when "happy" events are experienced by the infant, endorphins—"reward chemicals," the brain's natural opioids—are released. Endorphins encourage the growth and connections of nerve cells. Conversely, in animal studies, chronically high levels of stress hormones such as cortisol have been shown to cause important brain centres to shrink.

The neural circuits and neurochemistry of the brain develop in response to input from the environment. An infant with perfectly good eyes at birth would become irreversibly blind if he were confined to a dark room for five years, because the circuitry of vision needs the stimulation of light waves for its development. A "Darwinian" competition decides the survival of neurons and their synapses: those that get used survive and grow. Those deprived of the appropriate environmental stimulation atrophy or die, or fail to develop optimally.

A fundamental goal of human development is the emergence of a self-sustaining, self-regulated human being who can live in concert with fellow human beings in a social context. Vital for the healthy development of the neurobiology of self-regulation in the child is a relationship with the parent in which the latter sees and understands the child's feelings and can respond with attuned empathy to the child's emotional cues. Emotions are states of physiological arousal, either positive—"I want more of this"—or negative—"I want less of this." Infants and small children do not have the capacity to regulate their own emotional states, and hence are physiologically at risk for exhaustion and even death if not regulated by the interaction with the parent. Closeness with the parent, therefore, serves to preserve the infant's biological regulation.

Self-regulation requires the coordinated activities of anatomically separate brain areas, along with the benign dominance of the upper, more recently evolved regions of the brain over the lower ones. The oldest part of the brain—and the most essential for life—is the *brain stem,* where the primitive survival impulses of the "reptilian brain" arise and where basic autonomic functions are controlled, including—among others—hunger, thirst, cardiovascular and respiratory drives, and body temperature. The newest part of the human brain is the *neocortex* in the front of the brain. *Cortex* means "bark," as in the bark of a tree, and refers to the thin rim of grey matter enveloping the white matter of the brain. Made up largely of the cell bodies of nerve cells, or neurons, the cortex processes the most highly evolved activities of the human brain. This *prefrontal cortex* modulates our responses to the world not in terms of primitive drives but in terms of learned information about what is friendly, neutral or hostile and what is socially useful and what is not. Its functions include impulse control, social-emotional intelligence and motivation. Much of the regulating work of the cortex involves not the *initiation* of actions but the *inhibition* of impulses arising in the lower brain centres.

Mediating between the regulatory processes of the cortex and the basic survival functions of the brain stem is the *limbic* emotional apparatus. The limbic system includes structures located between the cortex and brain stem but also encompasses some parts of the cortex. The limbic system is essential for survival. Without it the regulatory and thinking capacities of the cortex would function like the brain of an idiot savant: intellectual knowledge would be disconnected from real knowledge of the world.

Emotions interpret the world for us. They have a signal function, telling us about our internal states as they are affected by input from the outside. Emotions are responses to present stimuli as filtered through the memory of past experience, and they anticipate the future based on our perception of the past.

The brain structures responsible for the experience and modulation of emotions, whether in the cortex or the midbrain, develop in response to parental input, just as visual circuitry develops in response to light. The limbic system matures by "reading" and incorporating the emotional messages of the parent. The centres of memory, both conscious and unconscious, rely on the interaction with the parent for their consolidation and for their future interpretations of the world. The circuits responsible for the secretion of important neurotransmitters like serotonin, norepinephrine and dopamine—essential for mood stability, arousal, motivation and attention—are stimulated and become coordinated in the context of the child's relationship with his caregivers. In the brains of infant monkeys, serious imbalances of these various neurochemicals have been measured after only a few days of separation from their mothers.

In the parent–child interaction is established the child's sense of the world: whether this is a world of love and acceptance, a world of neglectful indifference in which one must root and scratch to have one's needs satisfied or, worse, a world of hostility where one must forever maintain an anxious hypervigilance. Future relationships will have as their templates nerve circuits laid down in our relationships with our earliest caregivers. We will understand ourselves as we have felt understood, love ourselves as we perceived being loved on the deepest unconscious levels, care for ourselves with as much compassion as, at our core, we perceived as young children.

The disruption of attachment relationships in infancy and childhood may have long-term consequences for the brain's stress-response apparatus and for the immune system. A large number of animal experiments have established a powerful connection between early attachment disturbances and unbalanced stress-response capacities in the adult. The crux of this research is that disrupted attachment in infancy leads to exaggerated physiological stress responses in the adult. Obversely, nurturing attachment interactions in infancy provide for better modulated biological stress reactions in the adult.

For the satisfaction of attachment needs in human beings, more than physical proximity and touching is required. Equally essential is a nourishing emotional connection, in particular the quality of *attunement*. Attunement, a process in which the parent is "tuned in" to the child's emotional needs, is a subtle process. It is deeply instinctive but easily subverted when the parent is stressed or distracted emotionally, financially or for any other reason. Attunement may also be absent if the parent never received it in his or her childhood. Strong attachment and love exist in many parent–child relationships but without attunement. Children in non-attuned relationships may feel loved but on a deeper level do not experience themselves as appreciated for who they really are. They learn to present only their "acceptable" side to the parent, repressing emotional responses the parent rejects and learning to reject themselves for even having such responses.

Infants whose caregivers were too stressed, for whatever reason, to give them the necessary attunement contact will grow up with a chronic tendency to feel alone with their emotions, to have a sense— rightly or wrongly—that no one can share how they feel, that no one can "understand." We are speaking here not of a lack of parental love, nor of physical separation between parent and child, but of a void in the child's perception of being seen, understood, empathized with and "got" on the emotional level. The phenomenon of physical closeness but emotional separation has been called *proximate separation*. Proximate separation happens when attuned contact between parent and child is lacking or is interrupted due to stresses on the parent that draw her away from the interaction.

An example of such an attunement break occurs when the parent looks away first from the child during one of their intensely pleasurable eye-to-eye gaze interactions. Another attunement break occurs if the parent insists on stimulating a resting child because he (the parent) desires the mutual engagement, even if the child at that moment needs some respite from the intensity of their interaction.

"Primate experiments show that infants can undergo severe separation reactions even though their mothers are visually, but not psychologically, available," writes the UCLA psychologist, theorist and researcher Allan Schore. *"I suggest that proximate separations are a common and potent phenomenon in early personality development."*[8]

In *proximate separations* the parents are physically present but emotionally absent. Such parent–child interactions are increasingly the norm in our hyperstressed society. The levels of physiological stress experienced by the child during proximate separation approaches the levels experienced during physical separation. Proximate separation affects the young child on the unconscious physiological levels rather than on the conscious thought-feeling levels. It will not be recalled later as the adult looks back on his childhood experience, but it is entrenched as the biology of loss.

Experiences of proximate separation become part of the person's psychological programming: people "trained" in this way in childhood are likely to choose adult relationships that re-enact repeated proximate separation dynamics. They may, for example, choose partners who do not understand, accept or appreciate them for who they are. Thus the physiological stresses induced by proximal separation will also continue to be repeated in adult life—and, again, often without conscious awareness.

16

The Dance

of Generations

GIVEN THE INFORMATION PRESENTED IN previous chapters, it may seem as though parents are to blame for the later development of illness in their offspring. Such a conclusion is quite contrary to my intentions and entirely out of keeping with the scientific evidence. Parenting styles do not reflect greater or lesser degrees of love in the heart of the mother and father; other, more mundane factors are at play. Parental love is infinite and for a very practical reason: the selfless nurturing of the young is embedded in the attachment apparatus of the mammalian brain.

If a parent's loving *feelings* are constricted, it only because that parent has himself or herself suffered deep hurt. In my work with drug addicts in Vancouver's Downtown Eastside, I treat many substance-dependent men and women. Hardened as they are—with their criminal records, their continued drug-seeking, their HIV infections and their harassed and socially marginal lives—the deepest pain they all have is about the children whom they have abandoned or who have been taken from them. Without exception, they themselves were abused or abandoned in childhood.

Where parenting fails to communicate unconditional acceptance to the child, it is because of the fact that the child receives the parent's love *not as the parent wishes but as it is refracted through the parent's personality.* If the parent is stressed, harbours unresolved anxiety or is agitated by unmet emotional needs, the child is likely to find herself in situations of *proximate abandonment* regardless of the parent's intentions.

For better or worse, many of our parenting attitudes and responses have to do with our own experiences as children. That modes of parenting reflect the parent's early childhood conditioning is evident both from animal observations and from sophisticated psychological studies of humans.

Rhesus monkeys are a species of primates favoured by psychological investigators because of their relatively small size and ease of care. In a troop of these monkeys, about 20 per cent are "high reactors" who are more likely than others to exhibit depressive behaviours on separation from mother, along with greater and longer activation of the HPA axis, exaggerated sympathetic nervous system arousal and deeper suppression of immune activity. In human terms, we might call the high reactors temperamentally hypersensitive. Not unlike their human counterparts, they tend to end up at the bottom of the social hierarchy. Their offspring resemble them in behaviour, reactivity and social status.

Research has revealed that the "constitutional high-reactor destiny can be interrupted by changing the environment." The positive changes are passed on to future generations: "When reared with especially nurturing mothers, such animals show no signs of the usual behavioural disorder. Instead, they showed signs of precocious behavioural development and rose to the top of the hierarchy as adults. *Females adopted the maternal style typical of their especially nurturing mothers.*"[1]

These observations are not about learned behaviours, strictly speaking. For the most part, parent-child similarities in nurturing approach do not reflect cognitive learning, either in animals or in human beings. The intergenerational transmission of parenting style is largely a matter of physiological development, of how the limbic circuits of the brain become programmed in childhood and how the connections within the PNI super-system are established. As discussed in the previous chapter, the emotional brain of the child develops under the influence of the emotional brain of the parent. The child does not learn the parenting styles of his mother and father by imitation—or only in part. The biggest influence on the future parenting style of the child is the development of his emotional and attachment circuits in the context of his relationship with his parents. The same is true of the development of the child's stress-response apparatus.

One dramatic animal experiment will suffice to illustrate this principle. Tranquilizers like Valium and Ativan belong to a class of drugs called *benzodiazepines.* Like all pharmacological agents that affect mental functions, they work because certain brain areas have receptors for similar natural tranquilizing substances manufactured in the brain itself. The *amygdala,* an almond-shaped structure in the temporal lobe of the brain, is one of the main regulators of the fear and anxiety response. It is supplied with natural benzodiazepine receptors that, when activated, cool down our fearful reactions. Compared with adult rats who received less nurturing, in adult rats who had been licked and groomed more by their mothers *the amygdala was found to contain many more benzodiazepine receptors.* Maternal care in infancy influenced the physiology of anxiety regulation in the brain of the adult. These differences were not explained by genetic factors.[2]

Although the psychological development of humans is much more complex than that of animals, intergenerational transmission of parenting behaviour and of stress is also the general rule. It is similar to the development of the child's stress response. As a group of Canadian researchers have written, "Maternal care during infancy serves to 'program' behavioural responses to stress in the offspring *by altering the development of the neural systems that mediate fearfulness.*"[3] In short, anxious mothers are likely to rear anxious offspring, down through the generations.

Researchers developed scores assessing the quality of parent–child bonding. Scores of parental bonding were measured across three generations: between adult mothers and their mothers, and between these same adult mothers and their own daughters. The measures of bonding between mothers and daughters were consistent across the generations.[4]

In the adult children of Holocaust survivors with post-traumatic stress disorder (PTSD), disturbances of the HPA axis and cortisol production were found. The more severe was the parents' PTSD, the greater was the impairment in their children's cortisol mechanisms.[5]

Mary Ainsworth, an early associate of John Bowlby's and later professor of developmental psychology at the University of Virginia in Charlottesville, devised a method of assessing the pattern and quality of parent–child attachments. During the child's first year of life, researchers observed mother–infant interactions in the home, recording their perceptions. At one year, each infant–mother pair was brought into the laboratory for a brief experiment, called the Strange Situation. "At various times in the twenty-minute procedure, the infant stayed with the mother, with the mother and a stranger, with only the stranger, and alone for up to three minutes. The idea was (and still is) that separating a one-year-old from her attachment figure within a strange environment should activate the infant's attachment system. One should then be able to study the infant's responses at separation and reunion. The most useful assessments came at the reunion episode of this paradigm."[6]

The baby's response to the returning mother, it turned out, was programmed by how the mother had interacted with her during the first year of life. Those infants who had received attuned attention from their mothers at home showed signs of missing their mothers on separation. They greeted their returning mothers by initiating physical contact. They were soothed easily and returned quickly to spontaneous play. This pattern was called *secure*. There were also a number of insecure patterns, variously named *avoidant, ambivalent* or *disorganized*. Avoidant infants did not express distress on separating from the mother and avoided or ignored the mother on reunion. Such behaviour did not denote genuine self-reliance but the pseudo-autonomy that we noted, for example, in rheumatoid patients: the belief that they must depend only on themselves, since trying to obtain help from the parent was useless. Internally, however, these avoidant infants were physiologically stressed when the parent returned, as measured by heart rate changes. The infants falling into the insecure categories had been subjected to non-attuned parenting in the home. They had received implicit messages of maternal emotional absence, or mixed messages of contact alternating with distance.

Already at one year of age the infants were exhibiting relationship responses that would characterize their personalities and behaviours in the future. The Strange Situation experiment has been duplicated hundreds of times, in many countries. The observations at one year are accurate advance indicators of behaviour at adolescence, including such features as emotional maturity, peer relationships and academic performance. On all these measures, children who had been securely attached infants scored consistently better than insecurely attached ones.

However, as Daniel Siegel explains in his book *The Developing Mind,* the most crucial finding concerning the intergenerational transmission of parenting was that *the infant's performance in the Strange Situation could be accurately predicted even before the child was born.*

Professor Mary Main at the University of California, Berkeley, formerly a student of Dr. Ainsworth's, developed an accurate means of assessing an adult's childhood attachment relationship patterns with his parents. Her technique considers primarily not *what* a person said in response to questions but *how* he said it. The patterns of people's speech and the key words they "happen" to employ are more meaningful descriptors of their childhoods than what they consciously believe they are communicating. The intended meaning of words reflect only the speaker's conscious beliefs, from which painful memories are often excluded. The real story is told by the *patterns* of the narrative—fluent or halting, detailed or characterized by a paucity of words, consistent or self-contradicting, along with Freudian slips, revealing asides and apparent non-sequiturs.

The test developed by Mary Main is called the Adult Attachment Interview (AAI). Just as the responses of infants in the Strange Situations, the narratives of adults could also be classified along lines that reflected the degrees of security they had experienced in their early interactions with their parents.

It turns out that *"the AAI is the most robust predictor of how infants become attached to their parents."* In other words, what an adult unconsciously reveals about his own childhood during the course of the attachment interview will predict his own attachment patterns with his children. Thus, AAIs conducted with the parent *before the birth of an infant* was able to forecast accurately how the infant would behave in the Strange Situation at one year of life. Furthermore, when those children are followed two decades later, their performance in the Strange Situation is found to have accurately predicted their own patterns of narrative in the Adult Attachment Interview.

Thus, the adult's AAI narrative of his own childhood will often predict how he will nurture his future child, and therefore how his child, at one year, will respond in the Strange Situation. And, the child's behaviour in the Strange Situation will foretell the type of narrative she, in turn, will give about her childhood twenty years later!

Parenting, in short, is a dance of the generations. Whatever affected one generation but has not been fully resolved will be passed on to the next. Lance Morrow, a journalist and writer, succinctly expressed the multigenerational nature of stress in his book *Heart,* a wrenching and beautiful account of his encounters with mortality, thrust upon him by near-fatal heart disease: "The generations are boxes within boxes: Inside my mother's violence you find another box, which contains my grandfather's violence, and inside that box (I suspect but do not know), you would find another box with some such black, secret energy—stories within stories, receding in time."

Blame becomes a meaningless concept if one understands how family history stretches back through the generations. "Recognition of this quickly dispels any disposition to see the parent as villain," wrote John Bowlby, the British psychiatrist whose work threw scientific light on the decisive importance of attachment in infancy and childhood. Whom do we accuse?

If we see that stress is transmitted transgenerationally, we can better understand why so many of the histories we have encountered in this book speak of families with generations of disease or of several members of the same generation affected by widely disparate and apparently unrelated illnesses. Some random examples:

- •NATALIE: multiple sclerosis. Her oldest brother was an alcoholic who died of cancer of the throat. Her younger sister is schizophrenic. Her uncles and aunts were alcoholics. Her maternal grandfather was alcoholic. Her husband, Bill, died of bowel cancer. Her son has attention deficit (hyperactivity) disorder and has struggled with drug addiction.
- • VÉRONIQUE: multiple sclerosis. She believes she was conceived during an incestuous rape. In her adoptive family, the maternal grandfather was an alcoholic and her maternal grandmother developed Alzheimer's disease in her sixties. Among other medical problems, her father has early-onset high blood pressure.
- • SUE RODRIGUEZ: ALS. Her father died of alcoholic liver disease; one of her aunts died of a brain aneurysm, another in a house fire.
- • ANNA: breast cancer. Both her mother and maternal grandmother died of breast cancer—but neither through genetic transmission.

Anna inherited a breast-cancer gene on her father's side. She has two sisters: one is living with an alcoholic, the other is mentally ill.
- GABRIELLE: scleroderma, with features of rheumatoid arthritis. Her parents were alcoholics. Her brother has had a colectomy for cancer of the bowel, and her sister was recently diagnosed with breast cancer.
- JACQUELINE DU PRÉ: multiple sclerosis. Her grandmother was traumatized by the death of other children about the time her mother was born. Jacqueline's mother predeceased her with cancer, and her father developed Parkinson's disease.
- RONALD REAGAN: Colon cancer, Alzheimer's disease. His father and brother were alcoholics; his second wife developed breast cancer. His daughter died of metastatic malignant melanoma.

The reader may recall from chapter 1 the outraged letter from a rheumatologist in response to my article about Mary. I had suggested that Mary's childhood experiences of abuse and abandonment had created a coping pattern of repression and that her scleroderma was an outcome, in part, of that history. The specialist stated that scleroderma was an inherited disease, and that my arguments had "no credibility." She wrote, "This column has the effect of misinforming the lay public and falsely assigning responsibility for the development of scleroderma to the victims of this disease and to their families." We can now see that "assigning responsibility"—by which the rheumatologist meant allocating blame—is not the issue. The central issue is the unintentional transmission of stress and anxiety across the generations.

Another patient of mine, Caitlin, also died with scleroderma. Her course was much more rapid than Mary's, for she was dead less than a year after her diagnosis. I came to know Caitlin well only in her final months. Although I had delivered her children and remained their doctor, until her diagnosis with scleroderma she attended a female physician for her own medical problems.

Like Mary, Caitlin, too, was a kind and quiet soul with concern for everyone but herself. When she was asked how she was, her response was always accompanied by a warm, self-effacing smile that served to protect her listener from the physical and emotional pain she was experiencing. She would quickly divert the conversation to some matter of personal interest to the other, away from her own troubles.

I will not forget my last conversation with Caitlin, at her hospital bedside. Her lungs and heart were barely functioning; she was less than twenty-four hours from her death. I asked how she felt. She immediately turned her attention to me, inquiring what was happening in *my* life. I related, with some disappointment, that a weekly medical column I had been writing for a local newspaper had been, just that morning, cancelled by the editors. "Oh," she whispered, her face saddened with empathy, "how terrible that must be for you. You love writing so much." On the threshold of death from a disabling disease at age forty-two, leaving four children and a husband, she uttered not a word about how terrible she may have been feeling herself.

"It was a long-standing part of her nature to be cheerful and always welcoming, regardless of whether she was sick or well," her husband, Randy, told me in the course of a recent interview. According to Randy, Caitlin "bottled up a lot of emotion," particularly when she was upset. There were two items she would rarely talk about: her terminal illness and her childhood. "If she mentioned her childhood at all, it would be about the few good times that she had."

From Randy's perspective, there was every indication that the good times in his wife's childhood had been few and far between. Her father, a successful businessman, was a harsh and arbitrary taskmaster whose word was law. He was highly critical of Caitlin, the elder of the two children. "It seemed to me that she felt that when her parents conceived her, it was a great inconvenience. That she had come too soon and they really didn't want her."

That struck a chord with me. Caitlin had been a committed anti-abortion advocate but not the hostile or embittered kind. She knew that I supported women's right to decide whether to continue or abort their own pregnancy. Because we had a mutually respectful relationship, she once wrote me to urge that I stop referring patients to abortion clinics. In that letter she said, "If abortion had been legal at the time when I was a fetus, I would have been aborted." She had, said Randy, a deep feeling of not having been wanted.

Late in Caitlin's illness, an incident occurred that, in the telling, brought tears to Randy's eyes. "We were sitting here in the kitchen with all those pills she was supposed to be taking. She was feeling miserable. All of a sudden she burst out crying. She said, 'Oh, I wish I had a mother.' And her mother lived only a few blocks away. They were not emotionally close enough that the mom would come and comfort her and help her or put her arms around her. We had a homemaker at the time. She was there, cleaning the fridge. She felt so touched that she came over and hugged Caitlin. I thought, What a shame—this person who hardly knows her has more empathy for her than her own mother.

"But I don't want to blame the parents either. When you look at their family histories—well, her mother's dad walked out on his family when she was a little girl. She didn't have a dad, and her mom (Caitlin's grandmother) had to struggle on all alone."

Randy's view of Caitlin's childhood was confirmed in a subsequent interview with her brother. "There was little emotional support and love in the family," the brother said. "Our father was mean to us, and our mother was afraid. My mother is a very nice person—a great person—but she would never deal with the issues.

"My father was just overbearing. I don't think we could have been five or six years old when we were sent to the basement every Saturday to clean. We weren't allowed to come up until it was done. While we were at it, we would polish my father's army boots. They had to shine."

Caitlin, her brother said, was "a pretty gentle soul," but to her father "she was just stupid. The very fact that she went to university ticked him off. He had no respect for anything she did. She was in the La Leche League (a group that promotes breast-feeding). My father ridiculed that. 'How long is she going to breast-feed those kids—until they are teenagers?'"

After putting up with years of feeling dominated, even as an adult, this brother finally broke with his father and refuses to talk him. "Caitlin was very concerned that I had got myself out of the family. She couldn't understand why I had done that. I tried to tell her it was the best thing for me, that I was a better person for it. She didn't get it."

Caitlin's brother, too, wept as he recounted an incident identical to the one Randy had related. "Caitlin said to my wife on her deathbed, the day before she died—it's hard, those images—my wife sat with her and held her hand, and Caitlin said, 'I wish I had a mother like you.

I don't have a mother.' I think the world of my mother, but she wasn't a good mother. She wasn't loving."

The brother also revealed details of the family history that once more demonstrated the multigenerational nature of suffering. It was a shock to Caitlin and her brother to learn the truth of what had happened with their grandfather. An uncle who showed up for the funeral of Caitlin's grandmother informed them that the grandfather had not died when Caitlin's mother was a young child, which had been the family story, but had abandoned his wife and later divorced her.

All their lives, Caitlin and her brother had been told that their grandfather had passed away suddenly. "When we asked my mom what happened to her father, she always said, 'He died when I was seven years old of a heart attack.' Our grandmother had given us the same line. We were so upset because here was a grandmother whom we loved and thought the world of. To know the truth would have meant so much to us and to our relationship with her. But that's the way it always was. In our family you don't talk about difficult issues, you hide them."

Such lies, however innocently intended, never protect a child from pain. There is something in us that knows when we are lied to, even if that awareness never reaches consciousness. Being lied to means being cut off from the other person. It engenders the anxiety of exclusion and of rejection. In Caitlin it could only have reinforced the perception of not being wanted that flowed from her father's harshness and her mother's emotional absence.

Less than a year preceding the onset of her scleroderma, Caitlin suffered a major rejection at the hands of her family, having to do with her exclusion from the family business. "My sister was never in the calculations," her brother says. "It didn't seem abnormal at the time." Caitlin felt deeply hurt by the perceived rejection. She never brought up the matter to anyone, except to her brother shortly before her death. And she kept maintaining that he, the brother, should go back to the family. "She felt it was her obligation, her duty, to make things right. That would be the only thing Caitlin would do—to try to make things better."

Caitlin had been assigned a certain role in the family system, a role bequeathed to her by generations of family history. Her own mother was deprived of attuned parenting from an early age, since we can surmise that the family's problems did not begin the moment the grandfather abandoned his wife and children. We may be equally sure that the harsh parenting by Caitlin's father originated in his own troubled childhood. The combination of her parents' many unmet emotional needs led to Caitlin's desperation to make herself lovable and prepared her for the role of the kind, gentle, uncomplaining caregiver who never became angry and never asserted herself. That is how the child's adaptive responses to perceived parental demand, if repeated often enough, become character traits.

Caitlin adopted her assigned role successfully, but at the cost of her own health. The price was a lifetime of stress. Her role, and her life, ended with a rapidly fatal autoimmune illness within one year of a deep rejection that she no longer had the resilience to deal with.

Hans Selye, the founder of stress research, developed the concept of *adaptation energy.* "It is as though we had hidden reserves of adaptability, or adaptation energy, throughout the body. . . . Only when all of our adaptability is used up will irreversible, general exhaustion and death follow."[7] Aging, of course, is the normal process through which the reserves of adaptation energy become depleted. But physiologically stress ages us as well—as the language recognizes when people speak of "having aged overnight." Throughout her lifetime, much of Caitlin's adaptation energy had been diverted away from self-nurturing toward taking care of others. Her function had been determined by family dynamics during her childhood. By the time her illness struck, she had run out of energy.

Central to any understanding of stress, health and disease is the concept of *adaptiveness.* Adaptiveness is the capacity to respond to external stressors without rigidity, with flexibility and creativity, without excessive anxiety and without being overwhelmed by emotion. People who are not adaptive may seem to function well as long as nothing is disturbing them, but they will react with various levels of frustration and helplessness when confronted by loss or by difficulty. They will blame themselves or blame others. A person's adaptiveness depends very much on the degree of differentiation and adaptiveness of previous generations in his family and also on what external stressors may have acted on the family. The Great Depression, for example, was a difficult time for millions of people. The multigenerational history of particular families enabled some to adapt and cope, while other families, facing the same economic scarcities, were psychologically devastated.

"Highly adaptive people and families, on the average, have fewer physical illnesses, and those illnesses that do occur tend to be mild to moderate in severity," writes Dr. Michael Kerr.

> Since one important variable in the development of physical illness is the degree of adaptiveness of an individual, and since the degree of adaptiveness is determined by the multigenerational emotional process, *physical illness, like emotional illness, is a symptom of a relationship process that extends beyond the boundaries of the individual "patient."* Physical illness, in other words, is a disorder of the family emotional system [which includes] present and past generations.[8]

Children who become their parents' caregivers are prepared for a lifetime of repression. And these roles children are assigned have to do with the parents' own unmet childhood needs—and so on down the generations. "Children do not need to be beaten to be compromised," researchers at McGill University have pointed out.[9] Inappropriate symbiosis between parent and child is the source of much pathology.

The child's habitual adaptive responses to the family system give rise to the traits that, with time, become identified with her "personality." We have noted that personality does not cause disease—stress does. If we may speak of a disease-prone personality, it is only in the sense that certain traits—in particular, the repression of anger—increase the amount of stress in an individual's life. Now we see that concepts such as "the rheumatoid personality" or "the cancer personality" are misleading for yet another reason: they assume that an individual person is an isolated entity, not recognizing that he is situated in and shaped by a multigenerational family system. As Dr. Kerr suggests, it is much more illuminating to think of, say, a *cancer position* than a cancer personality. "The concept of a cancer personality, although certainly having some validity, is based in individual theories of human functioning. The concept of a cancer position is based in a systems theory of human functioning. In a family system the functioning of each person is influenced and regulated by the functioning of every other person."[10]

If individuals are part of a multigenerational family system, families and individuals are also parts of a much larger whole: the culture and society in which they live. The functioning of human beings can no more be isolated from the larger social context than can that of a bee in a hive. It is not enough, therefore, to stop at the family system as if it determined the health of its members without regard to the social, economic and cultural forces that shape family life.

Cancer and the autoimmune diseases of various sorts are, by and large, diseases of civilization. While industrialized society organized along the capitalist model has solved many problems for many of its members—such as housing, food supply and sanitation—it has also created numerous new pressures even for those who do not need to struggle for the basics of existence. We have come to take these stresses for granted as inevitable consequences of human life, as if human life existed in an abstract form separable from the human beings who live it. When we look at people who only recently have come to experience urban civilization, we can see more clearly that the benefits of "progress" exact hidden costs in terms of physiological balance, to say nothing of emotional and spiritual satisfaction. Hans Selye wrote, "Apparently in a Zulu population, the stress of urbanization increased the incidence of hypertension, predisposing people to heart accidents. In Bedouins and other nomadic Arabs, ulcerative colitis has been noted after settlement in Kuwait City, presumably as a consequence of urbanization."[11]

The main effect of recent trends on the family under the prevailing socio-economic system, accelerated by the current drive to "globalization," has been to undermine the family structure and to tear asunder the connections that used to provide human beings with a sense of meaning and belonging. Children spend less time around nurturing adults than ever before during the course of human evolution. The nexus previously based in extended family, village, community and neighbourhood has been replaced by institutions such as daycare and school, where children are more oriented to their peers than to reliable parents or parent substitutes. Even the nuclear family, supposedly the basic unit of the social structure, is under intolerable pressure. In many families now, both parents are having to work to assure the basic necessities one salary could secure a few decades ago. "[The] separation of infants from their mothers and all other types of relocation which leave few possibilities

for interpersonal contact are very common forms of sensory deprivation; they may become major factors in disease," wrote the prescient
Hans Selye.

In *Tuesdays with Morrie*, Mitch Albom reports that Morrie Schwartz,
his former professor terminally ill with ALS, "was intent on proving that
the word 'dying' was not synonymous with 'useless.'" The immediate
question is why one would have a need to prove this. No human being
is "useless," whether the helpless infant or the helpless ill or dying adult.
The point is not to prove that dying people can be useful but to reject
the spurious concept that people need to be useful in order to be valued. Morrie learned at a young age that his "value" depended on his
ability to serve the needs of others. That same message, taken to heart
by many people early in life, is heavily reinforced by the prevailing ethic
in our society. All too frequently, people are given the sense that they
are valued only for their utilitarian contribution and are expendable if
they lose their economic worth.

The separation of mind and body that informs medical practice
is also the dominant ideology in our culture. We do not often think
of socio-economic structures and practices as determinants of illness
or well-being. They are not usually "part of the equation." Yet the
scientific data is beyond dispute: socio-economic relationships have a
profound influence on health. For example, although the media and
the medical profession—inspired by pharmaceutical research—tire-
lessly promote the idea that next to hypertension and smoking, high
cholesterol poses the greatest risk for heart disease, the evidence is that
job strain is more important than all the other risk factors combined.
Further, stress in general and job strain in particular are significant contributors both to high blood pressure and to elevated cholesterol levels.

Economic relationships influence health because, most obviously,
people with higher incomes are better able to afford healthier diets,
living and working conditions and stress-reducing pursuits. Dennis
Raphael, associate professor at the School of Health Policy and
Management at York University in Toronto has recently published a
study of the societal influences on heart disease in Canada and elsewhere. His conclusion: "One of the most important life conditions
that determine whether individuals stay healthy or become ill is their
income. In addition, the overall health of North American society may

be more determined by the distribution of income among its members rather than the overall wealth of the society. . . . Many studies find that socioeconomic circumstances, rather than medical and lifestyle risk factors, are the main causes of cardiovascular disease, and that conditions during early life are especially important."[12]

The element of control is the less obvious but equally important aspect of social and job status as a health factor. Since stress escalates as the sense of control diminishes, people who exercise greater control over their work and lives enjoy better health. This principle was demonstrated in the British Whitehall study showing that second-tier civil servants were at greater risk for heart disease than their superiors, despite nearly comparable incomes.[13]

Recognizing the multigenerational template for behaviour and for illness, and recognizing, too, the social influences that shape families and human lives, we dispense with the unhelpful and unscientific attitude of blame. Discarding blame leaves us free to move toward the necessary adoption of responsibility, a matter to be taken up when we come in the final chapters to consider healing.

17

The Biology of Belief

THE SCIENTIFIC INSIGHTS OF BRUCE Lipton, a molecular biologist formerly at Stanford University in California, have profound implications for the understanding of illness, health and healing. In his public talks, as in personal interviews, he likes to throw his audience a scientific curve ball in the form of a question: "What is the brain of the individual cell?" The typical answer he receives, as he did from this interviewer, is: "The nucleus, of course."

Of course, the nucleus is *not* the *brain* of the cell. The brain is our organ of decision making, and it is the brain that acts as our interface with the environment. In the life of the individual cell, not the nucleus but the *cell membrane* fulfills the functions analogous to the activities of the brain.

In human embryological development, both the nervous system and the skin stem from the same tissue, the *ectoderm*. Individual cells use their membrane as both skin and nervous system. Like the skin, the membrane surrounds and protects the internal milieu of the cell. At the same time, it has on its surface the millions of molecular receptors that act as the cell's sensory organs: they "see" and "hear" and "feel" and—like the brain—interpret the messages arriving from the cell's external milieu. It also facilitates the exchange of substances and messages with the environment. The cell's "decision making" also takes place in the membrane and not in the nucleus, where the cell's genetic material is located.

As soon as we understand this fundamental biological reality, we are able to see past the popular assumption that genes are all-decisive in human behaviour and health. People may be forgiven for that misbelief. Expressions of near-religious awe from some scientists and politicians and prophecies of dramatic medical advances greeted announcements in 2000 that researchers were close to deciphering the human genome, the genetic blueprint for the human body. "Today we are learning the language in which God created life," then president Bill Clinton said at the White House ceremony marking the truce between two groups of scientists racing to complete the genome. "I truly feel this is going to revolutionize medicine because we are going to understand not only what causes disease but what prevents disease," enthused Dr. Stephen Warren, a U.S. medical geneticist and editor of *The American Journal of Human Genetics.*

The actual results of the genome project are bound to be disappointing. Although the scientific information uncovered is important for its own sake, very little can be expected from the genome program that will lead to broad health benefits in the near future, if ever.

First, there are many technical problems still to be solved. Our current state of knowledge about the genetic makeup of human beings may be likened to using a copy of *The Concise Oxford English Dictionary* as "the model" from which the plays of William Shakespeare or the novels of Charles Dickens were created. "All" that remains to duplicate their work now is to find the prepositions, grammatical rules and phonetic indications, then to figure out how the two authors arrived at their storylines, dialogues and sublime literary devices. "The genome is the biological programming," one of the more thoughtful science reporters wrote, "but evolution has neglected to provide even the punctuation to show where genes stop and start, let alone any helpful notes as to what each gene is meant to do."

Second, contrary to the genetic fundamentalism that currently informs medical thinking and public awareness, genes alone cannot possibly account for the complex psychological characteristics, the behaviours, health or illness of human beings. Genes are merely codes. They act as a set of rules and as a biological template for the synthesis of the proteins that give each particular cell its characteristic structure and functions. They are, as it were, alive and dynamic architectural and mechanical plans. Whether the plan becomes realized depends on far more than the gene itself. Genes exist and function in the context of living organisms. The activities of cells are defined not simply by the genes in their nuclei but by the requirements of the entire organism— and by the interaction of that organism with the environment in which it must survive. *Genes are turned on or off by the environment.* For this reason, the greatest influences on human development, health and behaviour are those of the nurturing environment.

Hardly anyone who raises plants or animals would ever dispute the primary role of early care in shaping how genetic endowment and potential will unfold. For reasons that have little to do with science, many people have difficulty grasping the same concept when it comes to the development of human beings. This paralysis of thought is all the more ironic, since of all animal species it is the human whose long-term functioning is most profoundly regulated by the early environment.

Given the paucity of evidence for any decisive role of genetic factors in most questions of illness and health, why all the hoopla about the genome project? Why the pervasive genetic fundamentalism?

We are social beings, and science, like all disciplines, has its ideological and political dimensions. As Hans Selye pointed out, the unacknowledged assumptions of the scientist will often limit and define what will be discovered. Settling for the view that illnesses, mental or physical, are primarily genetic allows us to avoid disturbing questions about the nature of the society in which we live. If "science" enables us to ignore poverty or man-made toxins or a frenetic and stressful social culture as contributors to disease, we can look only to simple answers: pharmacological and biological. Such an approach helps to justify and preserve prevailing social values and structures. It may also be profitable. The value of shares in Celera, the private company participating in the genome project, went up 1,400 per cent between 1999 and 2000.

The genome hype is not only poor science, it is also suspect as theology. In the Book of Genesis creation story, God fashions the universe first, then nature, and only afterwards does He shape humankind from the substance of the earth. He knew, even if Bill Clinton did not, that from their very earliest beginnings humans could never be understood apart from their environment.

The milieu of the human organism is the physical and psycho-emotional environment that shapes our development and affects our interactions with the world throughout the lifetime. The milieu of the individual cell is the cell's immediate surroundings, from which it receives messenger substances that originate in nearby cells, in nerve endings controlled from afar and in distant organs that secrete chemicals into the circulatory system. The information substances attach to receptors on the cell surface. Then, in the cell membrane—depending on how receptive the cell is at that moment—*effector* substances are produced that go to the nucleus, instructing the genes to synthesize particular proteins to carry out specific functions. These receptor-effector protein complexes— called *perception proteins*—Bruce Lipton explains, act as the "switches" that integrate the function of the cell with its environment:

> Although perception proteins are manufactured through molecular genetic mechanisms, *activation* of the perception process is "controlled" or initiated by environmental signals. . . . The controlling influence of the environment is underscored in recent studies on *stem cells.** Stem cells do not control their own fate. The differentiation of stem cells is based upon the environment the cell finds itself in. For example, three different tissue culture environments can be created. If a stem cell is placed in culture number one, it may become a bone cell. If the same stem cell was put into culture two, it will become a nerve cell, or if placed into culture dish number three, the cell matures as a liver cell. *The cell's fate is "controlled" by its interaction with the environment and not by a self-contained genetic program.*[1]

A key point in Dr. Lipton's astute explanation of biological activity is that at any one time, cells—like the entire human organism—can be either in defensive mode or growth mode but not both. Our perceptions of the environment are stored in cellular memory. When early environmental influences are chronically stressful, the developing nervous system and the other organs of the PNI super-system repeatedly receive the electric, hormonal and chemical message that the world is unsafe or even hostile. *Those perceptions are programmed in our cells on the molecular level.* Early experiences condition the body's stance toward the world and determine the person's unconscious beliefs about herself in relationship to the world. Dr. Lipton calls that process *the biology of*

---

* *Stem cells are multipotential embryonic cells that have not yet specialized into particular tissue types.*

belief. Fortunately, human experience and the ever-unfolding potential of human beings ensure that the biology of belief, though deeply physiologically ingrained, is not irreversible.

We have seen that stress is the result of an interaction between a *stressor* and a *processing system.* That processing apparatus is the human nervous system, operating under the influence of the brain's emotional centres. The biology of belief inculcated in that processing apparatus early in life crucially influences our stress responses throughout our lives. Do we recognize stressors? Do we magnify or minimize potential threats to our well-being? Do we perceive ourselves as alone? As helpless? As never needing help? As never deserving help? As being loved? As having to work to deserve love? As hopelessly unlovable? These are unconscious beliefs, embedded at the cellular level. They "control" our behaviours no matter what we may think on the conscious level. They keep us in shut-down defensive modes or allow us to open to growth and to health. We look now at some of these viscerally held perceptions more closely.

1. I have to be strong

As an artist and avid reader, Iris is highly intellectual. About ten years ago, at the age of forty-two, she was diagnosed with SLE (lupus). Iris grew up in Europe, immigrating with her family to the United States in her early twenties. Her father was tyrannical and unpredictable, and her mother, she reports, "did not exist separately from my father."

"I've thought about this theory of the body saying no when your mind can't," Iris says. "I've heard it before, and I have agreed with the principle before. I just don't like thinking of it in terms of me."

"Why not?" I ask her.

"It means you aren't strong enough . . . you're not capable of doing whatever it was to be strong enough." These words brought to mind an ovarian cancer patient who disliked my theory because, she said, it made her look like a "wimp."

"What if one truly isn't 'strong enough'?" I say. "If I tried to lift a ten-thousand-pound weight and somebody said, 'You're not strong enough for that,' I'd agree."

"Under those circumstances, I'd say, 'What are you, an idiot?'"

"That's the whole point. Sometimes the problem is not that we lack strength but that the demands we make on ourselves are impossible. So what's wrong with not being strong enough?"

The core belief in having to be strong enough, characteristic of many people who develop chronic illness, is a defence. The child who perceives that her parents cannot support her emotionally had better develop an attitude of "I can handle everything myself." Otherwise, she may feel rejected. One way not to feel rejected is never to ask for help, never to admit "weakness"—to believe that I am strong enough to withstand all my vicissitudes alone.

Iris quickly conceded that when her friends call her with their problems, she does not judge them or accuse them of being weak. They are comfortable relying on her and see her as empathic and supportive. It was clear that her double standard—higher expectations of herself than of others—had nothing to do with *strength*. It had to do with a lack of *power*, as experienced by the child. A child can be stronger than he should have to be, because he doesn't have power.

2. It's not right for me to be angry

Shizuko is forty-nine, the mother of two grown children. She was diagnosed with rheumatoid arthritis at twenty-one, shortly after arriving in Canada as a foreign student. Her birth mother died when she was four, after which her father married her aunt, her mother's sister. "My stepmother liked business more than she liked children," she says. Her father indulged all her material needs and desires but he was most often away from home.

Shizuko divorced her emotionally distant husband five years ago. "My marriage was terrible. When I was living with my husband, I was tired all the time, raising the kids. [Fatigue is a common symptom in the rheumatic diseases.] Before 3:00 p.m. I would lie on the couch, and my husband always complained, 'You did nothing, nothing.' He said I was using him to be a free meal ticket."

"Did you ever feel angry?"

"Yes, I was angry at him all the time."

"Did you express the anger?"

"No . . . The way my stepmother raised me, I think I am not supposed to be angry."

3. If I'm angry, I will not be lovable.

Alan, with cancer of the esophagus, has been unhappy in his marriage. The reader may recall his perception that his wife was unable to be "romantic, intimate and all the things that I need."

"How would you express your dissatisfaction? Do you ever get angry about it? Do you ever *feel* angry about it?"

"It's hard to relate because now I get angry all the time. We talk about it a lot more now."

"What happened to the anger before you were diagnosed with cancer?"

"I don't know. I see what you're getting at, and it's probably true."

"Where did you learn to repress anger?"

"That's a good one—I don't think I've analyzed this quite enough. I think it comes from a desire to be liked. If you're angry, people don't like you."

4. I'm responsible for the whole world

Leslie, a fifty-five-year-old social worker, also attributes his illness—in his case, ulcerative colitis—to the stresses of a relationship. "It began during my first marriage. There was a lot of stress, and that's when it was the worst. It hasn't been bad in a long time. Now I sometimes have some bleeding, but it is very limited.

"My relationship with my first wife was always up and down. I think she didn't want to be involved. It was never a partnership. I had to think for her. It got real crazy making, because I would have to think about what we could do together. She would never tell me what she wanted to do. I would have to come up with a movie that I thought we both would like, one we both could go, and be happy with."

"Didn't it upset you to play that role?"

"For sure."

"What did you do with that anger?"

"Swallowed it—no question. I couldn't fight because then she would say, 'You see, this is a bad marriage.' Conflict with her was considered an indicator that the relationship was bad.

"I had to be very, very careful. When I started going out with Eva, who is now my wife, and we would have a fight, I would start smiling. I told her I was enjoying that we could actually fight and be different, and she was not going to go away. I definitely had fears of people leaving, of abandonment."

It took Leslie several months after the initial onset of his symptoms to seek medical help. "I wasn't ready to accept my vulnerability in having problems. It had a lot to do with my perfectionism, wanting to be perfectly all right, to have nothing wrong with me."

When Leslie was nine years old, his father died suddenly of a heart attack, and two years later he witnessed the sudden death of his brother from a brain aneurysm. "After that, I had an obsessive ritual every night, a routine to make sure people would not die. 'Don't die, don't die . . .' It was my way of controlling people not dying in my life.

"One day, I was talking with my psychiatrist. I said, 'I gave up that ritual and I don't know where it went.' It was like an 'aha' experience— all of a sudden it came to me: 'I know where it went. I became a social worker, and now I'm trying to save the world!'

"It caused me a lot of stress when I was trying to save the world and wasn't succeeding. I was on stress leave two or three years ago. I finally recognized that I can't save the world. I even have a mantra that the psychiatrist and I came up with: 'I should be a guide, not a God.' It works for me."

"So you thought this entire unholy mess of a world out there was your fault?"

"At one point I believed that whether or not it was my fault, I was going to be the one to fix it."

"How did that manifest itself in your work?"

"Well, if my parents, I mean clients, were not doing well, I felt I didn't have enough knowledge. I needed to know more and have better skills. I needed to find the right solution, work harder, read more, go to workshops."

One did not have to search far for the meaning of Leslie's Freudian substitution of *parents* for *clients*. Not only did he become his mother's chief companion and solace after the deaths of his father and older brother, but it also turns out that he had been in that role from birth.

"My mom did want me to be happy. She was always concerned that I should be happy. That was something that I was always trying to do. I tried to be happy in my childhood. I didn't know what depression was; I didn't even know what sad feelings were.

"My mom used say I was such a good-natured child, which my brother wasn't. I was such a good-natured baby that she could wake me up in the middle of the night, play with me for a while and put me back, and I'd go back to sleep."

"Why on earth would she do that?"

"I guess she was lonely or needing some attention."

"So you had to work . . . from infancy."

"My mom's marriage with my father was terrible. They'd fight—it was bad before he died. It was my job to make her happy."

5. I can handle anything

Don, a fifty-five-year-old civil servant, had part of his colon removed for bowel cancer. Among his chronic stresses has been his compulsion to be hyperconscientious in his professional life. "Workload issues can make me angry," he says. "I don't know if *anger* is the right word, just *frustrated*. Not being able to handle just how much work I had on my desk at the time."

"What did you do about it?"

"I tensed up and calmed down by going for a walk, then came back and plunged back into the work and got it done."

"What about going to whoever is assigning the work and pointing out that it is too much for any one person to handle?"

"Never done that. I can handle anything, that's why. My determination was to be the one in the branch who handled the most files, in the best way."

"Why?"

"For a couple of reasons. One, competitive instincts. Two, I'm getting paid well, therefore I should do the best job. The approach I always took was, you give me the work and I'll do it. If you give me more work, I'll do more, and if you give me less work, I'll do less work."

"And when they cut back on staff and fewer people have to do the same amount of work?"

"I'd do more. In fact, what I'd often do is go to other people who were complaining about their workload and take work from them. There would always be a level of guilt that I could have done a better job on this or that file. There was always a little more I could do.

"I prided myself in presenting this image that I could do more than anyone else, in less time than anyone else."

"Any connections in that to your childhood?"

"Part of that was my mother. If I brought home a report card with three A's and three B's, it would be, 'Why not six A's?' Nothing I ever did was good enough. She always automatically assumed that I would become a professional of some sort. It was a big disappointment to my mother that I began my working life as a construction labourer."

6. I'm not wanted—I'm not lovable

Gilda Radner had a lifelong perception of not being wanted. An indication of the depth of Gilda's psychic despair came in some notes her husband, Gene Wilder, found after her death. In one, titled "Right-Hand Questions—Left-Hand Answers," the questions were written out in Gilda's right hand, the answers with the left. The technique and the title are especially significant: it is the right side of our brain, the holistic and emotional side, that controls the left hand. One right-hand question asks: "Is cancer your mother inside you?" The left-hand answer: "*She doesn't want me to exist* [her italics]."

7. I don't exist unless I do something. I must justify my existence

Joyce, the university professor with asthma, talked about her terrifying sense of emptiness when she was not busy doing something. I asked her what she meant by that.

"The emptiness is about this terror that if I don't fulfill things, demands, I won't really exist. As a child I was not part of the whole equation. All the tensions that were happening with my father and mother, and my father and brother, I was not part of. I was eight years younger, the daughter; I was the perfect little girl. All these things were going on. The feeling was that you don't exist unless you do something in the world."

8. I have to be very ill to deserve being taken care of

Angela was diagnosed two years ago with cancer of the uterus, at age forty-five. Prior to that, she had struggled with alcoholism, anorexia–bulimia, depression, and fibromyalgia. At one point she underwent intestinal bypass surgery for weight loss. She lost 150 fifty pounds within a year but soon gained it back, since neither her stress levels nor her eating habits had changed. I interviewed Angela at Hope House, a counselling and support centre in Vancouver for people with malignancy and other types of chronic disease.

"I feel like the cancer was a gift to me, because it got me out of Revenue Canada. I was an auditor for the past twelve years and I hated the job. Ever since childhood I've been unable not to take it personally when there is confrontation and conflict. People get upset when they are audited, and they project all their hate of government and taxes onto you. And I took it on."

"Why did it take cancer to get you out of a job that you hated and was bad for you?"

"I was depressed most of the time, and I felt like I had no choice. I've been working since I was seventeen. I knew that in other types of jobs, it would not be accepted to be sick so much. I was sick a lot. In the government, you're like a cog in the wheel. There are a hundred other people who do the same kind of thing that you do, so that if your work doesn't get done, they can shunt it off on someone else. That's the reason that I stayed there, out of fear."

"How did the cancer get you out of there?"

"After the cancer diagnosis, I began coming to Hope House and talking with the counsellors here. I was encouraged to take a look at my feelings and my life. I found out I've been trying to fit into something that I'm not really truly meant to be in."

"Did they tell you the title of my book?"

"Well, my body said no. I had major bleeding actually for two years, and they kept testing. They did two biopsies—on the second one they found cancer cells.

"When the doctor said the word *cancer* to me, my intuition, in a split millisecond, said Revenue Canada. It was pretty obvious to me. I've been having that message for the past twelve years, and I've been ignoring it."

"That's what I'm asking. Why did it take the cancer for you to do that?"

"Because it was *something real*. I've got this whole thing in my head that mood disorders are not enough. Bulimia is not enough. Everybody looks at disorders of the mind as, well, there's nothing wrong with you. There's a lot of judgment around."

"But there's a brain in there; it's a physical organ. Mood disorder is just as physiological as uterine cancer is."

"I agree with you. But that was my own judgment of it, because I believed what I had been conditioned to believe by my family and by society.

"Just the fact that I was depressed and that the job was making me sick was not enough, in my mind. I was so concerned about what other people would think—most important, my family."

The support system Angela has found since being diagnosed with cancer has enabled her to face her issues. "I have felt a safety I have never felt before," she says, "especially when I was going through all that stuff about detaching from Revenue Canada. And I've had a lot of encouragement to do things, loving things for myself, to do the things I have a passion for."

Although with human beings anything is possible, it would be hard to accept that Gilda's mother, Henrietta, truly did not want her daughter to exist, or that Leslie's mother ever consciously wished to make her son responsible for her happiness, or that Alan's parents wished to convey to him that he is only lovable when he is not angry. Most parents feel unconditional love for their children, and that is what they hope to get across to them. That is important to know, but it is not what matters. What matters are the child's unconscious perceptions, based on his innermost interpretations of his interactions with the world. Those interpretations, embedded at the cellular level, constitute the biology of belief that governs so much of what we feel, what we do and how we react to events.

A major contributor to the genesis of many diseases—all the examples we have looked at—is an overload of stress induced by unconscious beliefs. If we would heal, it is essential to begin the painfully incremental task of reversing the biology of belief we adopted very early in life. Whatatever external treatment is administered, the healing agent lies within. The internal milieu must be changed. To find health, and to know it fully, necessitates a quest, a journey to the centre of our own biology of belief. That means rethinking and recognizing—re-cognizing: literally, to "know again"—our lives.

Whichever modality of treatment people choose—conventional medicine with or without complementary healing; alternative approaches like energy medicine or various mind-body techniques; ancient Eastern practices like Ayurvedic medicine or yoga or Chinese acupuncture; the universal practice of meditation techniques; psychotherapy; nutritional healing—the key to healing is the individual's active, free and informed choice. There are many different ways to find that innate human capacity for freedom, outlined in many teachings, books and other sources. Liberation from oppressive and stressful external circumstances is essential, but that is only possible if we first liberate ourselves from the tyranny of our ingrained biology of belief.

18

The Power of

Negative Thinking

HE VANCOUVER ONCOLOGIST KAREN GELMON does not favour the war metaphors often applied to cancer. "The idea is that with enough might you can control, with enough might you can expel," she says. "It suggests that it's all a battle. I don't think that's a helpful way of looking at it. First, it's not valid physiologically. Second, I don't think it's healthy psychologically.

"What happens with our body is a matter of flow—there is input and there is output, and you can't control every aspect of it. We need to understand that flow, know there are things you can influence and things you can't. It's not a battle, it's a push–pull phenomenon of finding balance and harmony, of kneading the conflicting forces all into one dough."

What we might call the military theory of disease sees illness as a hostile force, something foreign that the organism must battle and defeat. Such a view leaves an important question unanswered, even in the treatment of acute infections where we are able to identify the micro-organisms invading the body and to kill them with antibiotics: *why will the same bacterium or virus spare one person but fell another?* An organism such as streptococcus, responsible for the so-called flesh-eating disease, lives in many people but triggers illness in only a few. Or it may be present in an individual at one time without leading to problems but mount a lethal attack at another time in the person's life. What accounts for the difference?

The nineteenth century saw a heated debate on this subject, conducted for decades between two outstanding figures in the history of medicine, the pioneer microbiologist Louis Pasteur and the physiologist Claude Barnard. Pasteur insisted that the virulence of the microbe decided the course of illness, Barnard that the vulnerability of the host body was most responsible. On his deathbed Pasteur recanted. *"Barnard avait raison,"* he said. *"Le germ n'est rien, c'est la terrain qui est tout."* [Barnard was right. The microbe is nothing, the ground (i.e., the host body) is everything.]

The dying Pasteur may have swung too far in the opposite direction, but perhaps he had an eye toward the future. Since his days, and especially with the coming of the antibiotic era in the mid-twentieth century, we have all but forgotten that the terrain for illness is a particular human being at a particular time of his life history. "Why does *this* patient have *this* disease *now?*" George Engel, a researcher of mind–body unity in medicine asked in 1977.[1] To all intents and purposes, modern medical practice has adopted a simplistic "cause-and-effect" perspective. When no obvious external agent is found—as is the case with most serious illnesses—it throws up its hands and declares the cause unknown. "Of unknown etiology" may be the most common phrase in textbooks of internal medicine.

While scientific humility is welcome, a cause-and-effect model of disease is itself a source of misperception. It cannot portray the ways that health is transmuted into illness or how illness may be turned toward health. Sufi tradition tells the famous story of the twelfth-century fool and sage, the mullah Nasruddin, on his hands and knees searching under a street light. "What are you looking for?" his neighbours ask. "My key," he replies. The neighbours all join in the search, carefully and systematically perusing every inch of ground in the vicinity of the lamp. No one finds the key. "Wait, Nasruddin," someone finally says, "just where did you lose this key?" "In my house." "Then why are you looking out here?" "Because, of course, I can see better here, under the light." It may be easier (and financially more rewarding) to research isolated causes such as microbes and genes, but as long as we ignore a broader perspective, diseases will always be of unknown etiology. A search outside where the light shines will not yield us the key to health; we have to look inside, where it is dark and murky.

No disease has a single cause. Even where significant risks can be identified—such as biological heredity in some autoimmune diseases or smoking in lung cancer—these vulnerabilities do not exist in isolation. Personality also does not by itself cause disease: one does not get cancer simply from repressing anger or ALS just from being too nice. A *systems model* recognizes that many processes and factors work together in the formation of disease or in the creation of health. We have demonstrated in this book a *biopsychosocial* model of medicine. According to the biopsychosocial view, individual biology reflects the history of a human organism in lifelong interaction with an environment, a perpetual interchange of energy in which psychological and social factors are as vital as physical ones. As Dr. Gelmon suggests, healing is a phenomenon of finding balance and harmony.

We cannot remind ourselves too often that the word *healing* derives from an ancient origin, meaning "whole"—hence our equation of wholesome and healthy. To heal is to become whole. But how can we be more whole than we already are? Or how is it that we could ever be less than whole?

That which is complete may become deficient in two possible ways: something could be subtracted from it, or its internal harmony could be so perturbed that the parts that worked together no longer do so. As we have seen, stress is a disturbance of the body's internal balance in response to perceived threat, including the threat of some essential need being denied. Physical hunger may be one such deprivation, but in our society the threat is most often psychic, such as the withdrawal of emotional nourishment or the disruption of psychological harmony.

"I cannot understand why I have cancer," one woman with ovarian cancer said. "I've led a healthy life, eaten well, exercised regularly. I've always taken good care of myself. If anyone should be a picture of health, it's me." The area she overlooked was invisible to her: the stress connected with emotional repression. Her conscientious (and conscious) best efforts to look after herself properly could not extend to an arena she did not know existed. That is why knowledge and insight have the power to transform, and why insight is more helpful to people than advice. If we gain the ability to look into ourselves with honesty, compassion and with unclouded vision, we can identify the ways we need to take care of ourselves. We can see the areas of the self formerly hidden in the dark.

The potential for wholeness, for health, resides in all of us, as does the potential for illness and disharmony. Disease *is* disharmony. More accurately, it is an *expression* of an internal disharmony. If illness is seen as foreign and external, we may end up waging war against ourselves.

The first step in retracing our way to health is to abandon our attachment to what is called positive thinking. Too many times in the course of palliative care work I sat with dejected people who expressed their bewilderment at having developed cancer. "I have always been a positive thinker," one man in his late forties told me. "I have never given in to pessimistic thoughts. Why should I get cancer?"

As an antidote to terminal optimism, I have recommended the power of negative thinking. "Tongue in cheek, of course," I quickly add. "What I really believe in is the power of *thinking*." As soon as we qualify the word *thinking* with the adjective *positive,* we exclude those parts of reality that strike us as "negative." That is how most people who espouse positive thinking seem to operate. Genuine positive thinking begins by including all our reality. It is guided by the confidence that we can trust ourselves to face the full truth, whatever that full truth may turn out to be.

As Dr. Michael Kerr points out, compulsive optimism is one of the ways we bind our anxiety to avoid confronting it. That form of positive thinking is the coping mechanism of the hurt child. The adult who remains hurt without being aware of it makes this residual defence of the child into a life principle.

The onset of symptoms or the diagnosis of a disease should prompt a two-pronged inquiry: what is this illness saying about the past and present, and what will help in the future? Many approaches focus only on the second half of that healing dyad without considering fully what led to the manifestation of illness in the first place. Such "positive" methods fill the bookshelves and the airwaves.

In order to heal, it is essential to gather the strength to think negatively. Negative thinking is not a doleful, pessimistic view that masquerades as "realism." Rather, it is a willingness to consider what is not working. What is not in balance? What have I ignored? What is my body saying no to? Without these questions, the stresses responsible for our lack of balance will remain hidden.

Even more fundamentally, *not posing those questions is itself a source of stress.* First, "positive thinking" is based on an unconscious belief that we are not strong enough to handle reality. Allowing this fear to dominate engenders a state of childhood apprehension. Whether or not the apprehension is conscious, it is a state of stress. Second, lack of essential information about ourselves and our situation is one of the major sources of stress and one of the potent activators of the hypo-thalamic–pituitary–adrenal (HPA) stress response. Third, stress wanes as independent, autonomous control increases.

One cannot be autonomous as long as one is driven by relationship dynamics, by guilt or attachment needs, by hunger for success, by the fear of the boss or by the fear of boredom. The reason is simple: *autonomy is impossible as long as one is driven by anything.* Like a leaf blown by the wind, the driven person is controlled by forces more powerful than he is. His autonomous will is not engaged, even if he believes that he has "chosen" his stressed lifestyle and even if he enjoys his activities. The choices he makes are attached to invisible strings. He is still unable to say no, even if it is only to his own drivenness. When he finally wakes up, he shakes his head, Pinocchio-like, and says, "How foolish I was when I was a puppet."

Joyce, the university lecturer with asthma, finds it impossible to say no. Her lungs say it for her. Joyce's fear of the no is not a fear of others but of an emptiness she feels when she is not pushing herself. "The emptiness," she says, "is about this terror that if I don't fulfill demands, I won't really exist." If she invoked her power of negative thinking, she could accept that fearsome void within herself. She would explore the experience of the void rather than attempt to fill it with positive deeds.

Michelle, diagnosed with breast cancer at age thirty-nine, used to seek relief in her lifelong habit of daydreaming. "No wonder I lived in a fantasy world," she said as she recalled her childhood unhappiness. "It's safer. You make up your own rules, and you can make it protective and as happy as you want it to be. The outside world is completely different."

One study conducted over nearly two years found that breast can-cer patients with a propensity to engage in pleasant daydreams had a poorer prognosis than their more reality-based counterparts. So did women who reported fewer negative feelings.[2]

According to a another report on women with recurrent breast can-cer, "Patients who reported little in the way of [psychological] stress . . . and who were rated by others as 'well adjusted,' were more likely to be dead at the one year follow-up."[3]

The repeated finding that people with happier, less troubled thought patterns can suffer more illness seems to defy common sense. The general belief is that positive emotions must be conducive to good health. While it is true that genuine joy and satisfaction enhance physical well-being, "positive" states of mind generated to tune out psychic discomfort lower resistance to illness.

The brain governs and integrates the activities of all organs and systems of the body, simultaneously coordinating our interactions with the environment. This regulating function depends on the clear recognition of negative influences, danger signals and signs of internal distress. In children whose environment chronically conveys mixed messages, an impairment occurs in the developing apparatus of the brain. The brain's capacity to evaluate the environment is diminished, including its ability to distinguish what is nourishing from what is toxic. People wounded in this way, as Michelle was during her childhood, are more likely to make decisions that lead to further stress. The more they tune out their anxiety via "positive thoughts," denial or daydreaming, the longer that stress will act on them and the more damaging it will be. When one lacks the capacity to feel heat, the risk of being burned increases.

Inevitably, negative thinking of the honest sort will will lead into areas of pain and conflict we have shunned. It cannot be otherwise. The overwhelming need of the child to avoid pain and conflict is responsible for the personality trait or coping style that later predisposes the adult to disease.

Natalie, with multiple sclerosis, put up with her alcoholic and emotionally abusive husband. She faithfully nursed him through his convalescence from two cancer operations and tolerated his petulant demands. He betrayed her, but even years after his death she cannot say no to other people's expectations. "Five years down the road and I still have not learned that I have to pace myself. My body says no to me frequently and I just keep going. I just don't learn." Natalie's explanation? "The nurse in me won't allow me to stop." That is the story she tells herself, as if there really existed a powerful "nurse" within her that controlled her behaviour. When Natalie does not say no, she is likely to find herself feeling stressed and suffer a flare-up of her MS. But to free herself from such stress she would have to accept the painful reality that only her own choices, based on childhood perceptions, render her incapable of asserting her needs.

Many people are blocked from self-knowledge and personal growth by the myth they feel compelled to hold on to, of having had a "happy childhood." A little negative thinking would empower them to see through the self-delusion that helps keep them stuck in self-harming behavioural patterns.

Jean, a thirty-five-year-old legal secretary, was diagnosed at age twenty-four with multiple sclerosis, having suffered weakness, dizziness, fatigue, bladder problems and, finally, a temporary loss of vision. She spent nearly a year in medical institutions, at an acute-care hospital and then at a rehabilitation facility. The few recurrences since then have been much milder.

Jean was married at nineteen. Her first husband was an older man, controlling and abusive. "Mostly emotional, verbal, but at the end physical. He hit me. That's when I left. He used to tape my phone conversations with my friends. I was working two jobs—playing music at night, daycare during the days. I handed over my paycheque. I didn't like working in his band. Too much travelling. I was lonely.

"I also had an eating disorder much of my life. When I went into hospital I weighted eighty-nine pounds, and I'm five foot six. I was anorexic. I left my husband one day and ended up in hospital the next."

"Your putting up for five years with an abusive older man could not have been accidental. I believe it says a lot about your family of origin."

"I could not disagree more. My family was the furthest thing from abusive you could possibly get. I have an incredibly supportive family. I have two brothers and a sister and parents who have been happily married for forty-five years. I was never treated with anything except care and love and tenderness."

"I didn't use the word *abusive* about your family. I said your story tells me a lot about your family of origin."

"Oh! [long pause] I don't know. What does it tell you?"

"Let me ask you first of all if you were ever sexually abused as a child."

"No, or . . . there was an episode of inappropriate touching when I was about eleven or so, by a fellow who worked with my dad somehow. We had a camp-out with people. I told my parents. *I didn't tell them at the time, I told them years later.*

"We were at a campfire, and I had shorts on. He was telling me what a pretty girl I was, and I was flattered. He was running his hand up the inside of my leg. I think the whole thing went on for about half an hour, but when he started touching me, that's when I made excuses and left. And I knew that I was upset about it.

"It's very cloudy to me. I was almost doubting myself. Even as I'm telling you, it seems like it was no big deal. But it stands out in my mind. I remember the feeling surrounding it, the dirty, bleh, horrible feeling surrounding it."

"If you had an eleven-year-old daughter and something like this happened to her, what would you like her to do?"

"Wow. I wouldn't like her to wait a couple of years until she said something, that's for sure."

"Why not?"

"Because I would want to be able to discuss it with her for starters, and help her to understand all the feelings she was feeling."

"And if she didn't tell you?"

"I would think that she was afraid to tell me. I don't know what I would think. . . ." Jean was holding back tears but wanted to continue with the interview.

"You recall your childhood as a happy one."

"Absolutely."

"Tell me about your anorexia."

"I think I was about fifteen. It never was labelled *anorexia* until later, when it developed into bulimia. I threw out my lunches and I never wanted my breakfast. I was so skinny. My parents worried a lot."

"Do you know what was in your mind?"

"Most of it was the insecurity around body image all teenage girls go through. I don't remember thinking that I was heavy—I never was. I just thought that I'd be more popular if I was skinnier. My self-worth was based on whether or not people liked me. I wanted everybody to like me."

"How it works, I believe, is that self-worth originates from how valued one feels by one's parents."

"I felt as though if I didn't get straight A's they wouldn't love me. I have an older sister who at that time was putting my parents through hell, and she was getting all the attention. My sister also had a bleeding disorder, so when we were younger a lot of the focus was on her. She was hospitalized, and they thought she had leukemia for the longest time."

"So let me run this past you again. You were a kid who unless she got A's felt unloved by her parents, who at age eleven was subjected to an inappropriate sexual advance. She felt sick about it but didn't tell her parents. At age fifteen you became anorexic. *And you had an absolutely happy childhood. What's wrong with this picture?*"

Jean laughs. "Well, because when I look back on my teenage years, it wasn't hell. It just wasn't. The eating disorder was just starting to assert itself. . . ."

"Do you notice you're avoiding my question?"

"What's wrong with that picture? That doesn't sound like a happy childhood to me. But I don't think about having an unhappy childhood."

Jean's exclusion of darker memories from recollections of childhood is typical. One study compared the perceptions of multiple sclerosis patients with those of non–MS controls. Subjects were asked to rate their home lives in childhood as unhappy, moderately happy or very happy.[4] Over eighty per cent in both groups said their home lives had been either moderately happy or very happy. It appears the vast majority in both groups, in roughly comparable proportions, remembered having grown up in the Land of Oz. But when people open up about their emotions and their lives, as Jean does here, such idealized images of childhood rarely remain intact.

"The anorexia was my way of not feeling my feelings. But as to why I dealt with it that way, I don't know."

"Perhaps you saw your parents as suffering with your sister, and you felt like protecting them. You took on the role of caregiver. You are likely still taking care of people, even when you aren't aware of it . . . your parents, your siblings or your husband."

"Or all of them. With my husband, if he is angry or upset, my first thought is, How do I fix it? And it's not even about me. It's automatic for me. Right now I'm working on curing his prostate cancer for him.* Aren't I clever?"

---

* Jean's husband, Ed, has been interviewed regarding his prostate cancer. See chapter 8.

"You're not going to do it. But you might work yourself into a flare-up."

"I did last year, when he was first diagnosed. And again, I had a flare-up when my husband's mother was ill and then died—I was so worried for him that I neglected looking after myself. I didn't eat right and I didn't rest enough. And I still do it with my parents. I shield them from all kinds of things that I fear would hurt them if they knew. I've never talked with them about the whole eating disorder. I don't always tell them if I have a flare-up of MS; I play it down because they worry so much."

Frequently an adult's recollections of life in her family of origin fail to take into account the hidden price the child had to pay for the parents' approval and acceptance. Pamela Wallin, the Canadian journalist diagnosed in 2001 with bowel cancer, provides a prime illustration of this in her memoir, *Since You Asked*. We see in her writing the split between the adult's recollections and the child's emotional reality. She cautions the reader early, "I'm warning you now. What follows may read like a travelogue for a town or a paid advertisement for the family, but as far as I am concerned, it's the truth. I feel I had a close-to-perfect childhood." It is impossible to reconcile that idealized view with some of the scenes Ms. Wallin (currently Canadian high commissioner in New York) candidly describes.

In one passage Pamela recalls being chronically intimidated by her older sister. Her suppressed rage over that reached such a boiling pitch that once she vindictively wounded her sister on the arm. "Bonnie still carries the scar on her arm from a wound I inflicted deliberately just a day before a big date on which she was to wear a new sleeveless dress. She had to borrow a shawl to hide the unsightly act of revenge." To this day, Ms. Wallin writes, she blames Bonnie for instilling in her a fear of the dark. To get rid of Pamela when her boyfriend was visiting, Bonnie chased her younger sibling into the bedroom, turned off the light switch and slammed the door. "She knew full well I would be too scared of potential monsters under the bed to make my way across the room in the dark and turn the light back on, so it all but guaranteed I would stay shuddering out of her way for the remainder of the evening." The story is told with a touch of joviality.

At work here is a kind of "false memory syndrome" in reverse: on the conscious level, people often remember only the happy parts of childhood. Even if troubling incidents are recalled, the emotional aspects of those events are suppressed. Parental love is legitimately remembered, but the child's feelings of not being understood or supported emotionally are not. In this case, absent is any recollection of how a child might feel who lacks the safety of confessing to her parents her terror and rage at repeatedly being imprisoned alone in a dark room. This lack of safety was confirmed by a more painful episode that occurred in Pamela's adolescence, when she did seek her mother's help and intervention regarding a troubling situation in the classroom. Pamela's mother was a teacher in the school her daughters attended. "Only once did she chastise me. One of our grade-school teachers was fondling our budding breasts during class, and Mom was reluctant to believe my charges against one of her respected colleagues. She said, and I suppose it reflected the times, that I should explain to the other girls that we should sit in such a way as to make his unwanted groping impossible. We did and simply waited for year's end so we would move on to the next grade and out of his reach. . . . But we all seemed to survive the experience without emotional scars." The problem is in the "seem[ing] to survive." Emotional scars are most often invisible. But scars of any type are less strong and less resilient than the tissue they replace: they remain potential sites of future pain and disruption, unless they are recognized and tended to.

An oblique remark in her book that "kids often find it impossible to talk to their parents openly" is Pamela's only reference to not having been heard as a child. There is no depiction of the frustration a child feels when the significant adults do not know how to listen. In general, she insists that she had no "personal demons to exorcise," a remark exemplifying the denial of anxiety, anger and negative emotion that the studies on cancer patients have consistently reported.

Tuning out—by, say, daydreaming—enables the child to endure experiences that otherwise may trigger reactions that would land him in trouble. This kind of dissociation is in play when a person retains conscious recall for events in the past but not for their traumatic emotional resonance. It explains many "happy childhoods," such as Iris with SLE insists she had, despite her father's tyranny and the emotional absence of her mother.

"My father had a very short leash on his temper, and when he got angry, you never knew what was going to happen. Dishes could fly, somebody might get kicked."

"Did you get kicked?"

"Never. I was my father's favourite."

"How did you achieve that status?"

"*I disappeared.* I developed that ability early in life."

"Do you remember feeling unhappy as a child?"

"Unhappy? No."

"Could a child in those circumstances not feel sad or unhappy about things?"

"You get numb, usually."

"So you don't really know if you felt unhappy or sad because you would have numbed it out."

"That's right. I don't remember huge blocks of my childhood."

"Why would someone have to numb out? Why couldn't you just go to somebody and talk about it? What about your mom?"

"Well, no, I couldn't talk to my mother because I didn't want her to know I was unhappy, for one thing. For another, she didn't really exist as a separate entity apart from my father. She was a neutral person.

"A child has very little language. I was numb, but on the other hand I was quite happy in my numbness."

"Oh?"

"I played with dolls . . . okay, never mind about that . . . I was going to say I *chewed* dolls!"

"What do you mean you chewed them?"

"They were made out of plastic, and I'd chew their fingers and toes!"

"You were mutilating them, in your suppressed rage. Consider this—when do we have to numb things out?"

"When you're in pain . . ."

"Eventually when you numb it out enough, you can imagine that you're happy. You are only happy because you numbed out a huge part of your reality. Which is to say that you're not really living life to the fullest at all."

"Agreed."

———

Finally, I come back to Darlene, the insurance broker whose ovarian cancer was diagnosed inadvertently, during an infertility investigation. Nothing in her history could be described as even remotely painful. The only negative experience in her life, as she recounted it, has been her ovarian cancer and its unexpected recurrence despite diagnosis and treatment at a very early stage. The initial prognosis, she said, had been "celebratory," the recurrence "devastating."

"I've always wanted to be in control of my life, have always taken care of myself. I eat well, exercise, I'm in great shape. I've never had any bad habits." The one risk factor she did have was infertility. Darlene describes her life in terms that, to my ears, sound too good to be true. In all her childhood she cannot recall one single unhappy incident, not one moment of fear, anger, anxiety or sorrow.

"I'm the oldest of three girls. The three of us are incredibly close, as are my mom and dad, who are still living and very healthy. On top of that, my husband's family and I are very close. I have been blessed with family and have also been blessed with really good, deep friends—some that I've had since I was five years old. My friends and family have been a huge source of inspiration. I think I've been very lucky in that respect."

Darlene's cancerous right ovary was removed in 1991. She retained her left one, hoping to become pregnant in the future. She did successfully conceive a year later.

"We all talk about that five-year mark, and I made it through that. It was about five and a half years after my oophorectomy, and my son was four, when I had what I considered very innocuous symptoms: I was tired, I had lost a little bit of weight—but only five pounds, nothing major. I had a toddler, a career and a busy household. My lower back was sore, but again I thought I was struggling with a toddler, trying to get him in and out of snowsuits.

"When I was diagnosed again in 1996, and it had metastasized, we were obviously devastated—and the prognosis was very, very different, with spread to the other ovary, the uterus and spots in the lower abdomen."

"I'm curious, given the past history of ovarian cancer, why these symptoms did not alarm you sooner. What might you have advised a friend with your history and your symptoms?"

"Oh, well. When it comes to my friends, if they have an ingrown toenail, I send them to a gynecologist."

"This difference in how you treat yourself and how you treat others is one of the hints you've given me that not all in your life may have been as you picture it. Another is when you said, 'I think I've been very lucky,' in describing your relationships. The *I think* is a qualifier—to me it indicates uncertainty; it reflects an internal debate. Perhaps what you think is not what you feel; otherwise, you simply would have asserted that you feel fortunate.

"I also note that you smile when you talk about your pains and aches, as if you're trying to soften the impact of your words. How and why might you have learned to do that? The reflex of smiling when people talk about physical pain, or about painful events or incidents or thoughts I see all the time. Yet when infants are born, they have no capacity to hide feelings whatsoever. If an infant is uncomfortable or unhappy, she'll cry, show sadness, show anger. Anything that we do to hide pain or sadness is an acquired response. It may make sense to hide negative emotion in some circumstances, but so many of us do it all the time, and we do it automatically.

"Somehow people are trained—some more than others—into unknowingly taking care of other people's emotional needs and minimizing their own. They hide their pain and sadness, even from themselves."

Darlene listened thoughtfully. She neither agreed nor disagreed. "It's an interesting perspective. We should definitely bring it up in my ovarian cancer support group. I don't know how to respond to it right now, and I don't believe you really need an immediate response. It is intuitive and very thought-provoking. I thank you for that."

Developing the courage to think negatively allows us to look at ourselves as we really are. There is a remarkable consistency in people's coping styles across the many diseases we have considered: the repression of anger, the denial of vulnerability, the "compensatory hyperindependence." No one chooses these traits deliberately or develops them consciously. Negative thinking helps us to understand just what the conditions were in our lives and how these traits were shaped by our perceptions of our environment. Emotionally draining family relationships have been identified as risk factors in virtually every category of major illness, from degenerative neurological conditions to cancer and autoimmune disease. The purpose is not to blame parents or previous generations or spouses but to enable us to discard beliefs that have proved dangerous to our health.

"The power of negative thinking" requires the removal of rose-coloured glasses. Not blame of others but owning responsibility for one's relationships is the key.

It is no small matter to ask people with newly diagnosed illness to begin to examine their relationships as a way of understanding their disease. For people unused to expressing their feelings and unaccustomed to recognizing their emotional needs, it is extemely challenging to find the confidence and the words to approach their loved ones both compassionately and assertively. The difficulty is all the greater at the point when they have become more vulnerable and more dependent than ever on others for support.

There is no easy answer to this dilemma but leaving it unresolved will continue to create ongoing sources of stress that will, in turn, generate more illness. No matter what the patient may attempt to do for himself, the psychological load he carries cannot be eased without a clear-headed, compassionate appraisal of the most important relationships in his life.

As we have seen, *it is not others' expectations and intentions but the perception we have of them that serves as the stressor.* Jean, with MS, was driven into a flare-up by worrying about her husband's prostate cancer and assuming responsibility for his seeking the proper medical care. Ed resented Jean's "controlling" him but was unable to communicate his feelings to her. Jean's belief that she needed to be responsible for Ed—and Ed's belief that she was out to control him—were perceptions based on relationship templates each constructed as young children.

"Most of our tensions and frustrations stem from compulsive needs to act the role of someone we are not," wrote Hans Selye. The power of negative thinking requires the strength to accept that we are not as strong as we would like to believe. Our insistently strong self-image was generated to hide a weakness—the relative weakness of the child. Our fragility is nothing to be ashamed of. A person can be strong and still need help, can be powerful in some areas of life and helpless and confused in others. We cannot do all that we thought we could. As many people with illness realize, sometimes too late, the attempt to live up to a self-image of strength and invulnerability generated stress and disrupted their internal harmony. "I can handle anything" was how Don, with bowel cancer, described his pre-illness stance. "I couldn't try to help all the women with ovarian cancer," Gilda Radner realized after her recurrence, "and I couldn't read every letter I received because it was tearing me apart."

If we learn to think negatively, we stop minimizing our emotions of loss. Many times in the interviews for this book people qualified their hurts and stresses by words and phrases such as "just a little bit" or "maybe" or "might have." Recall Véronique, with multiple sclerosis, who dismissed the cumulative stresses of a breakup with an alcoholic boyfriend, financial destitution and other difficult life events as "not necessarily bad."

Do I live my life according to my own deepest truths, or in order to fulfill someone else's expectations? How much of what I have believed and done is actually my own and how much has been in service to a self-image I originally created in the belief it was necessary to please my parents? Magda, with severe abdominal pain, became a physician against her own inclinations—not because her mother and father overtly demanded or even requested it, but because she had made their beliefs into her own. And she did this long before she was old enough to decide what to do with her life. "Almost all my accomplishments were in one way or another connected not to *my* aspirations, but to the aspirations of my father," wrote Dennis Kaye, dying of ALS.

"[I am] not half the woman my mother had been," wrote former U.S. first lady Betty Ford. "My mother was a wonderful woman, strong and kind and principled, and never let me down. She was also a perfectionist, and tried to program her children for perfection."[5] The strength to think negatively would have allowed Mrs. Ford to ask herself how kind it really is to try to "program" a child for perfection. Instead of fleeing from her self-judgments into alcoholism and a lifetime of stress that culminated in breast cancer, had she been armed with some negative thinking, Betty would have rejected the impossible standards of perfectionism. "I am not half the woman my mother had been," she might have said with glee, "and I don't even want to be a quarter of the woman she was. I just want to be myself."

Laura, with ALS, felt guilty because she did not want bed-and-breakfast guests while her housekeeper was on vacation. She took on the task of hosting because her fear of guilt was greater than her fear of the stress of looking after guests while disabled.

"I try to help people all the time," said Ed, with prostate cancer. And if not? "I feel bad about it. Guilty." For many people, *guilt is a signal that they have chosen to do something for themselves.* I advise most people with serious medical conditions that there is probably something out of balance if they do *not* feel guilty. They are still putting their own needs, emotions, interests last. The power of negative thinking could permit people to *welcome* their guilt rather than shun it. "I feel guilty?" Ed could say. "Wonderful. Hallelujah! It means I must have done something right, acted on my own behalf for a change."

"The biggest thing is the control factor," Ed said about his wife Jean's solicitous mothering of him. "I'm resentful." And how does he deal with it? "I hide it." The power of negative thinking could enable Ed to accept the guilt of asserting himself against his wife's interference with his personal decisions, no matter how well meant. A therapist once said to me, "If you face the choice between feeling guilt and resentment, choose the guilt every time." It is wisdom I have passed on to many others since. If a refusal saddles you with guilt, while consent leaves resentment in its wake, opt for the guilt. Resentment is soul suicide.

Negative thinking allows us to gaze unflinchingly on our own behalf at what does not work. We have seen in study after study that compulsive positive thinkers are more likely to develop disease and less likely to survive. Genuine positive thinking—or, more deeply, positive *being*—empowers us to know that we have nothing to fear from truth.

"Health is not just a matter of thinking happy thoughts," writes the molecular researcher Candace Pert. "Sometimes the biggest impetus to healing can come from jump-starting the immune system with a burst of long-suppressed anger."[6]

Anger, or the healthy experience of it, is one of the seven A's of healing. Each of the seven A's addresses one of the embedded visceral beliefs that predispose to illness and undermine healing. We look at them in our final chapter.

19

The Seven A's

of Healing

BOTH THE ONSET OF MALIGNANT melanoma and the body's ability to survive it involve the immune system. Despite the potentially fatal prognosis, there are many recorded cases of spontaneous remission in this disease—the cancer disappears without medical treatment. Although it accounts for only 1 per cent of all cancers, malignant melanoma provides for 11 per cent of spontaneous cancer remissions.[1]

The journal *Cancer* reported a case of spontaneous healing in a seventy-four-year-old man. His cancer was found in a suspicious-looking mole removed from his chest wall in 1965; he experienced a recurrence seven years later, also on his chest, in the form of numerous small moles. The new lesions resulted from local spread of his original melanoma. However, this time the patient refused all further treatment. Eight months later a follow-up visit showed that the small tumours that had seeded the area were flatter and lighter in colour. The patient permitted a small biopsy to be performed; there was pigmentation at the site but no cancer. The following year further clinical signs of healing were present.

The immunologic findings were illuminating. Three things happened: first, lymphocytes had attacked the tumour; then, larger cells called macrophages literally helped to eat up the melanoma; finally, there was an influx of antibodies that also participated in destroying the malignancy. This man's body had mobilized formidable immune resources to defeat the cancer.

Spontaneous remission raises two important questions: why, in some people, are such resources not powerful enough to destroy cancerous cells in the first place, before the clinical development of melanoma; and what enables the immune system in some people to overcome this potentially deadly cancer even after it does arise? We have asked the same questions regarding the highly differing outcomes from one person to another of other diseases, despite the apparent similarities of the pathologies involved.

In a series of three studies, researchers in San Francisco looked at the Type C pattern of repressed negative emotion in melanoma patients. During an eighteen-month follow-up, they found a strong correlation between repression and the likelihood of relapse or death. Natural killer cells attack abnormal cells, thus providing a line of defence against cancer. NK cells have a demonstrated capacity to digest melanomas. As in breast cancer, they are less active in emotionally repressed individuals.

One of the studies examined the thickness of the original melanoma in relationship to personality. Thickness of the cancer at first biopsy is correlated with prognosis: the thicker the lesion, the less favourable the outlook. Higher scores on the Type C Melanoma Coping scale were found to be associated with thicker lesions: "Type C Melanoma Coping is characterized by patients' acceptance of having melanoma, having more concern for family members than for themselves, trying not to think about it, coping by perseverance and trying to keep busy, keeping feelings inside, and being considered strong and capable at handling things."[2]

These San Francisco findings confirmed the conclusions of an earlier 1979 study, that melanoma patients who had a harder time adjusting to the diagnosis—in other words, whose responses were less accepting and resigned—were also less likely to suffer relapse.[3]

Even rudimentary psychological support can make a difference suggests a pilot study conducted at the UCLA, School of Medicine, by the psychiatrist F. I. Fawzy. Thirty-four people with comparable stage 1 melanoma were enrolled in the experimental and control arms of the study, respectively. "Fawzy's intervention was strikingly minimal. It consisted of only six structured group sessions over a 6-week period, with each session lasting 1 1/2 hours. The group meetings offered (1) education on melanoma and basic nutritional advice; (2) stress management techniques; (3) enhancement of coping skills; and (4) psychological support from the staff and from other group members." Six years later, ten of the original thirty-four patients of the group that had not received psychological support had died, and three others had had recurrences. In the support group, only three of the thirty-four had died, four had experienced recurrences.[4] Earlier in the study, improved immune function had been demonstrated among the patients in the support group.[5]

It would stand to reason that people with melanoma and other cancers would enhance their ability to reverse the malignant process if they were helped to understand themselves and to become more self-accepting and assertive in their emotional coping styles. Harriette, a fifty-year-old writer, is convinced that her decision to fight the cancer her own way, including with intensive psychotherapy, is responsible for the remission of the malignant melanoma on her right shin.

"I didn't trust doctors much. I did some research and found this alternative clinic in Tijuana. They treated melanoma as a whole-body condition, which was the first thing I liked. Surgery on the leg and nothing to follow up didn't feel right to me. I went to Mexico, and they treated me with a whole series of things, including a vaccine, diet, tonic and some herbal pastes that they use to burn it off the leg. I went back every month, and then three months and six months, but I started realizing that there was something wrong with the way I was handling things. For starters, I didn't have a GP in Canada. I resisted the authority of doctors, yet here I was accepting treatment from doctors in Mexico.

"I thought at least I should get a GP—and that is actually when I met you. You didn't know me from Adam, but as soon as I mentioned melanoma, you said, 'You know there is a psychological profile for melanoma patients, don't you?' Nobody had ever mentioned it to me before, but when you described it, I completely fitted the picture. You also told me that I should have the surgery and you could arrange it, but that surgery by itself might not help unless I also dealt with my inability to feel my own feelings and with all the other problems.

"So I did therapy for six months. It was very intense. After that, I had the surgery. The plastic surgeon was shocked to see me, because he told me that the biopsy he had originally taken showed that I'd had invasive malignant melanoma, quite advanced, quite deep. He expected the worst. And yet, when he did the surgery, he found that it was just abnormal pigmented tissue but no longer melanoma."

I wondered whether it was the treatment in Mexico or the therapy Harriette underwent that had made the difference. Although I was unfamiliar with the details of the Mexican regimen, it had likely included the BCG vaccine to stimulate the immune system—an approach that, in some cases, has been successfully used against melanoma. Harriette believes it was a combination of everything. "I do think that the treatment in Mexico was working, but the thing kept tingling, and I kept feeling there was something still there—a tingling and a darkening under the skin."

"What did you find out in therapy?"

"I had to go back right to the beginning. My mother died when I was a toddler. I was the middle one of three sisters all under four, two of us in diapers. My younger sister was just eight months old and very colicky. None of us got much attention but what little there was my sister got. We were shuffled around from place to place, because my father was a travelling salesman. Within a year he married somebody who looked a lot like my mother. She was the Wicked Witch of the West. She had her own problems. She was awful to us. Finally, she sent us away to a French-Canadian convent.

"She didn't like children—she was the eldest of fourteen children and had raised all her younger brothers and sisters. She couldn't wait to get out of her home. She rose to be a secretary at the Canadian embassy in Costa Rica. She was a very bright woman, but at thirty-three she was becoming a spinster. My father apparently asked every available woman in the English-speaking community of Costa Rica to marry him within the year after my mom's death, and they all said no. She said yes—she didn't want children, she didn't like children, but that was her pact with the devil. And my dad? He was at home fifty-two days the first year they were married. Here she was with three little girls who had all these communicable diseases, one after the other, quarantined. I certainly see her side of it.

"I remember copying out French poems and leaving them outside the bathroom door when she was in there having a shower. She never, ever responded to them. She never acknowledged them."

"So you were trying very hard to bring her into a relationship with you."

"Yes, and it never worked. . . . My sisters were terrified of her. She locked herself up in her bedroom and would leave us with the maids. I remember when we needed something—and this is a scene that happened over and over again—the three of us would sneak up to her bedroom door and practice trying to say "M . . ." Finally after standing there for twenty minutes or however long it was and not having the courage—not one of us—to say "Mommy," we would sneak away again.

"The sense was that we couldn't ask for anything. That's what I learned. I learned not to need or want, not to ask because it wasn't there, and when we did, we were ridiculed.

"One of my earliest memories is from around age three or four—sitting in a dress by myself playing with a doll. I was fine playing, but the sense was that there was no connection. There was nobody around; I was completely isolated. This was safe, but there wasn't a sense of happiness, only that I had figured out how to protect myself."

"By being alone."

"By being alone and yes . . . without feeling contact.

"There are other fragments that come up. For a long time I've had this image of lying in what felt like clouds; I was on a bed of clouds with a grey and colourless sky above me and this one ray of sun hitting me, but it was cold. The sense of really being completely alone, that even this ray, which might be love, wasn't. I saw that learning not to feel was what I had to do in order to survive."

Such experiences—or the conclusions Harriette drew from them—left her isolated in life, or in relationships that, she felt, depleted her more than they nurtured her. Her intensive therapy was aimed at developing emotional competence. Emotional competence is the capacity that enables us to stand in a responsible, non-victimized, and non-self-harming relationship with our environment.* It is the required internal ground for facing life's inevitable stresses, for avoiding the creation of unnecessary ones and for furthering the healing process. Few of us reach adult age with anything close to full emotional competence. Recognizing our lack of it is not cause for self-judgment, only a call for further development and transformation.

Pursuing the seven A's of healing will help us grow into emotional competence.

---

* See chapter 3.

1. Acceptance

Acceptance is simply the willingness to recognize and accept how things are. It is the courage to permit negative thinking to inform our understanding, without allowing it to define our approach to the future. Acceptance does not demand becoming resigned to the continuation of whatever circumstances may trouble us, but it does require a refusal to deny exactly how things happen to be now. It challenges the deeply held belief that we are not worthy enough or "good" enough to be whole.

Acceptance also implies a compassionate relationship with oneself. It means discarding the double standard that, as we have seen, too often characterizes our relationship with the world.

As a physician, I have seen much human suffering. It may be futile, attempting to select one patient who has suffered in more ways than any of the others. Yet were I pushed to such a choice, I know immediately which patient that would be. Her story never made it into any of the chapters in this book; her illnesses would have put her in almost every chapter. I will call her Corinne. She's in her early fifties and has had the following diagnoses: Type II diabetes, morbid obesity, irritable bowel syndrome, depression, coronary vascular disease with two heart attacks, high blood pressure, lupus, fibromyalgia, asthma and—most recently—cancer of the bowel. "I have enough medication," Corinne says, "that I don't have to have breakfast; I just have to take all the pills. There are thirteen pills at breakfast time alone."

Corinne was my patient for twenty years. Much of what I learned, I learned from her, and from my other patients who, like Corinne, shared their stories with me. As a child, Corinne experienced every sort of boundary deprivation and violation one can imagine. As an adult, she has been a chronic caregiver not only to her husband, children, siblings and friends but to anyone brought into her home. Until recently, saying no has been impossible. It is still painful even now, despite her dire health status and despite the fact that she can only get around by means of a motorized scooter.

"I see myself as a big blob. There is no shape. I can see people's auras. Mine looks black and grey, and there is no definition. It's like you're looking at someone in the fog, and you can sort of see part of an outline, but nothing whole."

"If you saw somebody else who had difficulty establishing boundaries, would you dismiss them as a big blob?"

"No. I know several people who are overweight and I don't classify
them as big blobs. It's more my own self-image of who I am as a person.
I feel like Jell-O when it comes to emotional things."

"So who's talking to me now? Is this the big blob talking to me? Is
there no sense of somebody real at home?"

"I guess maybe a little bit. I can't say 100 per cent, no."

"Let's just look at that 'little bit,' then."

"The little bit wants to be in control and not allow other people to
decide and make decisions for her without her consent."

"What more can you say about yourself? What are your values?"

"That I don't sleep around, I don't cheat and I don't lie and I obey
the law of the land and I try to be the best person that I can be to
other people."

"Is that only because you don't know how to say no, or is it genuine
caring?"

"It's both. The majority is genuine caring."

"So how can you say you're just a big blob?"

"Because I'm Jell-O when it comes to saying no to my mother.
Only a few days ago I couldn't say to her, 'No, it would be better for
you to come in the summer, not now.' I couldn't say that to her. I wasn't
willing to make the decision."

"If somebody else told you that they had difficulty making such a
decision, what would you say?"

"I'd say that you have a lot of difficulty telling your mom what you
want to tell her . . . and that you need to be stronger."

"Without necessarily telling them what to do, what would you
understand about them?"

"I would understand they're scared that if they assert themselves,
they're going to be rejected."

"If you cannot say that about yourself, it's only because are not
paying the kind of compassionate attention to yourself that you would
automatically grant somebody else. You cannot force yourself to say no
if you don't know how to. *But at least you can give compassionate attention
to the individual who is having trouble saying no.*

"Let's look at the bind you put yourself in," I continued. "On one hand, you don't know how to say no; on the other hand, you condemn and judge yourself for not being able to say no. You end up calling yourself a big blob. With compassionate attention, you will see yourself as clearly as you see that other person—as someone who's scared. And you will say that not as a judgment but as a compassionate observation— *that person is really scared. That person is really hurt.* She has—*I have*—a hard time saying no, because that brings up the immediate risk of rejection.

"You can't force yourself to say no any more than you can force someone else to say no, but you can be compassionate toward yourself."

"I would hold someone else's hand to help them say no—but I wouldn't hold my hand to help me say no."

"And if they didn't know how to say no, you'd still accept them. You'd say.'Look, I understand that it's really hard for you—you're not ready.'"

"But I don't say that about myself—I get angry at myself."

"The thing that would help you the most, I believe, is that quality of compassionate attention toward yourself. You can work on that."

"Will it give me back the energy that I seem to be feeling is zapped from me?"

"So much of your energy goes into looking after others, and so much of what remains goes into self-judgments. Being this harsh on yourself takes up a lot of energy.

"The objective fact is that you're facing many serious medical problems. You are at risk—there's no question about it. I don't know how things will go. But with all that you have to deal with, the more compassionate you can be toward yourself, the more able you are to give yourself the best possible chance."

Compassionate curiosity about the self does not mean liking everything we find out about ourselves, only that we look at ourselves with the same non-judgmental acceptance we would wish to accord anyone else who suffered and who needed help.

2. Awareness

All those seeking to heal—or to remain healthy—need to reclaim the lost capacity for emotional truth-recognition, which is wonderfully illustrated by the neurologist Oliver Sacks in his book *The Man Who*

Mistook His Wife for a Hat. Sacks relates an anecdote about a group of aphasic patients responding to a televised address by then-president Ronald Reagan.

Aphasia—from the Greek *a* (for "not") and *pha* ("to speak")—is the loss of the ability to speak or to understand spoken language. It is the result of focal brain damage, as from a stroke. "There he was, the old Charmer, the Actor, with his practised rhetoric, his histrionisms, his emotional appeal—and all the patients were convulsed with laughter. Well, not all: some looked bewildered, some looked outraged, one or two looked apprehensive, but most looked amused. The President was, as always, moving—but he was moving them, apparently, mainly to laughter. What could they be thinking? Were they failing to understand him? Or did they, perhaps, understand him all too well?"[6]

Sacks's aphasic patients were reacting to Reagan's unconscious expressions of Emotion II—tone, body language, facial mannerisms. They found his emotions incongruent with his spoken message: in other words, they saw through his dissembling, conscious or unconscious. They read the emotional reality, not the word-reality Reagan was able to conjure up in his own mind and that he was so adept at conveying to those who, like him, were themselves emotionally shut down. *"Either he is brain-damaged or he has something to conceal,"* one of Sacks's patients said. Recall the words of Reagan's biographer: *He feels the opposite of what he says.*

Animals and young humans are highly competent at picking up on real emotional cues. If we lose that capacity as we acquire language, it is only because we receive confusing messages from our immediate world. The words we hear tell us one thing, the emotional data say something different. If the two are in conflict, one will be repressed. In the same way, when a child's eyes diverge, the brain will suppress images from one eye in order to avoid double vision. The suppressed eye, unless corrected, will become blind. We repress our emotional intelligence in order to avoid an ongoing war with the crucial people in our lives, a war we cannot possibly win. And so we lose our emotional competence even as we gain verbal intelligence. Aphasiacs, it would appear, go through the reverse process. Much as a blind person will develop an extraordinary capacity to hear, the aphasiac develops an enhanced ability to perceive emotional reality.

"People are usually no better than chance at detecting lies from a liar's demeanour, even when clues to the deceit are evident from facial expression and tone of voice," a group of psychiatric researchers reported in *Nature* magazine in May 2000. "People who can't understand words are better at picking up lies about emotions."

Full awareness would mean that we would regain our lost capacity to perceive emotional reality and that we are ready to let go of the paralyzing belief that we are not strong enough to face the truth about our lives. There is no magic to it. The blind person learns to pay more attention to sound than the sighted. The aphasiac learns to notice his internal reactions to words, since the cognitive parts of the brain can no longer tell him what the message is. Those internal reactions, gut feelings, are what we lost as we "grew up."

Clearly, we do not need to lose language skills in order relearn emotional perception. To develop awareness, though, we do have to practise, pay constant attention to our internal states and learn to *trust* these internal perceptions more than what words—our own or anyone else's—convey. What is the tone of voice? The pitch? Do the eyes narrow or open? Is the smile relaxed or tight? How do we feel? *Where do we feel it?*

Awareness also means learning what the signs of stress are in our own bodies, how our bodies telegraph us when our minds have missed the cues. In both human and animal studies, it has been observed that the physiological stress response is a more accurate gauge of the organism's real experience than either conscious awareness or observed behaviour. "The pituitary is a much better judge of stress than the intellect," Hans Selye wrote. "Yet, you can learn to recognize the danger signals fairly well if you know what to look for."

In *The Stress of Life*, Selye made a compilation of physiological danger signals. He listed physical signs such as pounding of the heart, fatigue, sweating, frequent urination, headaches, backaches, diarrhea or dryness of the mouth; emotional signs such as emotional tension or overalertness, anxiety, loss of joie de vivre; and behavioural expressions such as unusual impulsivity or irritability and a tendency to overreact. We can learn to read symptoms not only as problems to be overcome but as messages to be heeded.

3. Anger

"I never get angry," a Woody Allen character says in one of his movies, "I grow a tumour instead." Throughout this book we have seen the truth of that droll remark in numerous studies of cancer patients. We have also seen that the repression of anger is a major risk factor for disease because it increases physiological stress on the organism.

Not only does the repression of anger predispose to disease but the experience of anger has been shown to promote healing or, at least, to prolong survival. People with cancer who have been able to muster anger at their physicians, for example, have lived longer than their more placid counterparts. In animal experiments the expression of anger has been found to be less physiologically stressful than the suppression of it. In rats who fight others when caged together, slower growth of tumours has been found than in more docile animals.

Studies apart, we have seen that every one of the interviewees in the previous chapters acknowledged difficulties around the communication of anger, no matter what their disease or condition. "The way my stepmother raised me, I think I'm not supposed to be angry," said Shizuko, with rheumatoid arthritis. "I was short-circuiting my visceral expression of anger," said Magda, with severe abdominal pain.

Here the issue of anger becomes confusing and raises many questions. How can we encourage people to be angry when we see that children suffer from their parents' outbursts? In many of the patient histories we have seen a similar pattern: a raging parent, a repressed child. Should Magda's father have suppressed his anger? "I kept thinking of all the times my father raised his voice," said Donna, whose brother Jimmy died of malignant melanoma. "I remembered his voice and the screaming and the yelling, and I thought, This is not how you should live. This is not what we should have experienced."

On the surface, it seems like a paradox. If the expression of anger is "good," Magda's father and the father of Jimmy and Donna were only acting in a healthy fashion. Yet the effect of their anger was corrosive to their children's self-concept and health. Suppressing anger may have negative consequences, but should we encourage its expression if it harms others?

The mystery only deepens. Not only is the unbridled outpouring of anger harmful to the recipients or bystanders but it can also be deadly to the one who rages. Heart attacks can follow upon outbursts of rage. In general, high blood pressure and heart disease are more likely to happen in persons who harbour hostility. A study of nearly two hundred men and women conducted at the Johns Hopkins School of Medicine, Baltimore, in 2000 found that hostility and a drive for dominance were "significant independent risk factors for coronary heart disease."[7] A great volume of research has connected hostility with high blood pressure and coronary disease.

As we can readily deduce by now, the relationship between rage and cardiovascular disease is also a function of the psycho-neuro-immune apparatus. The sympathetic nerves are activated in rage states. Narrowing of the blood vessels occurs with excessive sympathetic flight-or-fight activity, increasing the blood pressure and decreasing oxygen supply to the heart. The hormones secreted during the stress response in rage states raise lipid levels, including serum cholesterol. They also activate clotting mechanisms, further heightening the risk of blockages in the arteries.

"It was blind rage, I was sure, that had gotten me into this fix with my heart, as well as genetics," wrote the journalist Lance Morrow in his memoir of heart disease. The blind rage that later triggered Morrow's heart attacks was the volcanic eruption of the anger a child learned to repress in his family of origin.

How then to resolve the dilemma of anger? If the expression of anger is harmful and so is its repression, how do we hope to attain health and healing?

The repression of anger and the unregulated acting-out of it are both examples of the *abnormal release of emotions* that is at the root of disease. If in repression the problem is a lack of release, acting out consists of an equally abnormal suppression of release alternating with unregulated and exaggerated venting. I had a fascinating conversation on these two seemingly opposite ways of coping with Allen Kalpin, a physician and psychotherapist in Toronto. He points out that both repression and rage represent *a fear of the genuine experience of anger.*

I found Kalpin's description of genuine anger surprising, even as it rang completely true to me. His explanation made me realize the confusion in our commonly received ideas about this emotion. Healthy anger, he says, is an empowerment and a relaxation. The real experience of anger "is physiologic experience without acting out. The experience is one of a surge of power going through the system, along with a mobilization to attack. *There is, simultaneously, a complete disappearance of all anxiety.*

"When healthy anger is starting to be experienced, you don't see anything dramatic. What you do see is a decrease of all muscle tension. The mouth is opening wider, because the jaws are more relaxed, the voice is lower in pitch because the vocal cords are more relaxed. The shoulders drop, and you see all signs of muscle tension disappearing."

Dr. Kalpin's mode of therapy works along the lines first developed by Dr. Habib Davanloo of McGill University, Montreal. Davanloo made a practice of videotaping his clients during therapy encounters so that they themselves could see their bodily manifestations of emotion. Kalpin, too, tapes some of his psychotherapy sessions.

"In a tape of one of my clients, he describes powerful surges of electricity going through his body—and he talks about them as they're happening—but outwardly he's just sitting there describing it. If you're watching the tape without the sound on, you'll see a person looking quite focused and quite relaxed, but you wouldn't necessarily even guess that the person was angry."

If anger is relaxation, what then is rage? When I am in a rage, my face is tight, my muscles are tense and I am sure I look anything but relaxed. Here Dr. Kalpin makes a crucial distinction. "The question is, What do people really experience when they experience rage? It's fascinating to ask people. If you really ask, the majority of people will describe anxiety. If you ask in physical, physiologic terms what they are experiencing in their body when they feel rage, for the most part, people will describe anxiety in one form or another."

"It's true," I said, "tightening of the voice, shallow breathing, muscle tension are signs of anxiety, not of anger."

"Exactly. Their anger is not physiologically experienced, it is only being acted out."

Acting out through bursts of rage is a defence against the anxiety that invariably accompanies anger in a child. Anger triggers anxiety because it coexists with positive feelings, with love and the desire for contact. But since anger leads to an attacking energy, it threatens attachment. Thus there is something basically anxiety-provoking about the *anger experience,* even without external, parental injunctions against *anger expression.* "Aggressive impulses are suppressed because of guilt, and the guilt exists only because of the simultaneous existence of love, of positive feelings," says Allen Kalpin. "So, the anger doesn't exist in a vacuum by itself. It is incredibly anxiety-provoking and guilt-producing for a person to experience aggressive feelings toward a loved one."

Naturally, the more parents discourage or forbid the experience of anger, the more anxiety-producing that experience will be for the child. In all cases where anger is completely repressed or where chronic repression alternates with explosive eruptions of rage, the early childhood history was one in which the parents were unable to accept the child's natural anger.

If a person unconsciously fears the power of his aggressive impulses, there are various forms of defence available to him. One category of defence is discharge, by which we regress to an early childhood state when we dealt with the intolerable buildup of anger by acting it out. "You see, the acting-out, the yelling, the screaming and even the hitting, all that a person does, serves as a defence against the experience of the anger. It's a defence against keeping the anger inside where it can be deeply felt. Discharge defends against anger being actually experienced."

The other way we can avoid the experience of anger is through repression. So repression and discharge are two sides of the same coin. Both represent fear and anxiety, and for that reason, both trigger physiological stress responses regardless of what we consciously feel or do not feel.

The paralyzing difficulty many people have with anger toward loved ones is illustrated repeatedly in the interviews we have seen. Jean, unable to tell her parents about being molested at age eleven, idealizes her relationship with them rather than acknowledge her anger. Her husband, Ed, has a corrosive resentment toward what he regards as controlling behaviour from his wife but cannot experience anger openly and directly. Jill, with ovarian cancer, is upset with her doctors for having missed the diagnosis but not at her husband, Chris, for having failed to notice her pain and weight loss over several months. Leslie, with ulcerative colitis, "swallowed" his anger toward his first wife. "No question about it. I couldn't fight because then she would say, 'You see, this is a bad marriage.'" He is delighted to find himself in a marriage now where the experience of anger does not threaten the relationship.

The anxiety of anger and other "negative" emotions like sadness and rejection may become deeply bound in the body. Eventually it is transmuted into biological changes through the multiple and infinitely subtle cross-connections of the PNI apparatus, the unifying nexus of body/mind. This is the route that leads to organic disease. When anger is disarmed, so is the immune system. Or when the aggressive energy of anger is diverted inward, the immune system becomes confused. Our physiological defences no longer protect us or may even turn mutinous, attacking the body.

"It may prove valuable to regard cancer less as a disease than as a disorder in the body's biochemical signals," writes the psychotherapist Luis Ormont, who has worked with mobilizing people's anger in group therapy with cancer patients. "To alter these signals is to produce an impact on the body's immunological defenses. It would follow that any form of intervention designed to restore the body to physical health must use more than physical means. Since emotions dramatically influence the biochemical system, one way of providing immunotherapy is by giving psychotherapy to patients."[8]

People diagnosed with cancer or with autoimmune disease, with chronic fatigue or fibromyalgia, or with potentially debilitating neurological conditions, are often enjoined to relax, to think positively, to lower their stress levels. All that is good advice, but impossible to carry out if one of the major sources of stress is not clearly identified and dealt with: the internalization of anger.

Anger does not require hostile acting out. First and foremost, it is a physiological process to be experienced. Second, it has cognitive value—it provides essential information. Since anger does not exist in a vacuum, if I feel anger it must be in response to some perception on my part. It may be a response to loss or the threat of it in a personal relationship, or it may signal a real or threatened invasion of my boundaries. I am greatly empowered without harming anyone if I permit myself to experience the anger and to contemplate what may have triggered it. Depending on circumstances, I may choose to manifest the anger in some way or to let go of it. The key is that I have not suppressed the experience of it. I may choose to display my anger as necessary in words or in deeds, but I do not need to act it out in a driven fashion as uncontrolled rage. Healthy anger leaves the individual, not the unbridled emotion, in charge.

"Anger is the energy Mother Nature gives us as little kids to stand forward on our own behalf and say *I matter,*" says the therapist Joann Peterson, who conducts workshops on Gabriola Island, in British Columbia. "The difference between the healthy energy of anger and the hurtful energy of emotional and physical violence is that anger respects boundaries. Standing forward on your own behalf does not invade anyone else's boundaries."

4. Autonomy

Illness not only has a history but also *tells* a history. It is a culmination of a lifelong history of struggle for self.

From a simple biological perspective, it may appear that the survival of the physical organism ought to be nature's ultimate goal. It would seem, however, that the existence of an autonomous, self-regulating psyche is nature's higher purpose. Mind and spirit can survive grievous physical injury, but time and again we see that the physical body begins to succumb when psychic integrity and freedom are jeopardized.

Jason has been an insulin-dependent diabetic since he was five. *Diabetes mellitus* derives its name from the Greek for "sweet urine," for in this disease excess sugar is filtered by the kidneys from the bloodstream into the urine. In diabetes the gland cells of the pancreas are unable to produce enough insulin, the hormone required to help sugar from digested food to enter the cells. Apart from the immediate physiological risks of high glucose levels, diabetes involves potential damage to many organs of the body.

Now twenty-three, Jason is blind in his right eye from diabetes-induced vascular injury. He also suffers from weakened cardiac muscles, a leaking heart valve and malfunctioning kidneys. At times he is unable to walk, owing to a reversible nerve inflammation called diabetic neuropathy. Jason and his mother, Heather, were my patients for about ten years. In the past twelve months, he has had to be rushed to emergency repeatedly for medical crises including heart failure and meningitis. He may not have many more years to live. According to his internal medicine specialist, his prognosis is "guarded."

Heather is in a chronic state of anxiety and exhaustion mingled with resentment, which she believes are due to Jason's stiff-necked refusal to take care of himself when it comes to eating the right kinds of food, paying close attention to his insulin requirements, attending medical appointments and having a healthy lifestyle. Of course, for a mother, the stakes are high. Her experience has been that when she does not take charge, Jason becomes ill. She has lived many years with the very real possibility that were she to relax her guard, even for a day, Jason could end up in a coma, or worse.

His most recent hospitalization followed a several-week bout of vomiting that left him weak, dehydrated and in convulsions. Heather was by his bedside one day when Jason had another seizure. "Nurses, residents and specialists came running," she relates. "Jason's eyes were rolling backward, and his arms and legs were shaking. They were injecting medications through the IV in his arm when he sat straight up, opened his eyes and looked straight at me. In a loud voice he said, 'Let go!' But I can't let go. I will not let my son die."

Jason does not recall the incident. "I must have been really out of it," he says.

"Any idea what you might have meant?" I ask.

"The first thing that springs to mind is just to let me go. My saying 'let me go' would not have meant to let me die, just 'stop being so overbearing. Let it go. Let me do what I'm going to do.' It's my life. I'll make my mistakes, but my mom has got to let me do that. Being diabetic and having somebody else try to control me has been such a large part of my life."

Whatever his mother's motivation, and no matter how much he has manipulated her into taking care of him, Jason's salient experience is of a lack of autonomy. He has had no capacity to assert himself openly. His yearning for an autonomous self and his anger towards his mother have taken the form of resistance—including resistance toward his own physical health. "It was always like suffocation," he told Heather. "No matter what I did, it seemed to be wrong. When I said 'let go,' it would have meant 'just back off. Let me live the way I'm going to live. I'm going to live my way, and of course I'm going to make mistakes—everybody does. I never felt free to make my own mistakes."

If there is one lesson to draw from the history of Jason and Heather, as from all the personal stories and all the studies we have considered in this book, it is that people suffer when their boundaries are blurred. By treating Jason all his life like a child for whom she must assume all responsibility, Heather has helped to hold him back from real personhood. By reacting like a child, Jason has held himself back.

In the final analysis, disease itself is a boundary question. When we look at the research that predicts who is likely to become ill, we find that the people at greatest risk are those who experienced the most severe boundary invasions before they were able to construct an autonomous sense of self. In 1998, *The American Journal of Preventive Medicine* published the results of the Adverse Childhood Experiences (ACE) study. There were over ninety-five hundred adult participants in this research project. Childhood stressors such as emotional or sexual abuse, violence, drug use or mental illness in the family were correlated with adult risk behaviours, health outcomes and death. There was a "strong graded relationship" between dysfunction in the family of origin and adult health status—that is, the greater the exposure to dysfunction had been in childhood, the worse the health status was in the adult and the greater were the chances of untimely death from cancer, heart disease, injury or other causes.[9]

Most commonly in the lives of children, boundaries are not so much violated as simply not constructed in the first place. Many parents cannot help their child develop boundaries because they themselves were never enabled to do so in their own formative years. *We can only do what we know.*

Without a clear boundary between himself and his parent, the child remains enmeshed in the relationship. That enmeshment is later a template for his way of connecting to the rest of the world. Enmeshment—what Dr. Michael Kerr called a lack of differentiation—comes to dominate one's intimate relationships. It can take two forms, withdrawal and sullen and self-defeating resistance to authority, like Jason's, or chronic and compulsive caretaking of others, like Heather's. In some people the two may co-exist, depending on with whom they happen to be interacting at the moment. Since the immune confusion that leads to disease reflects a failure to distinguish self from non-self, healing has to involve establishing or reclaiming the boundaries of an autonomous self.

"Boundaries and autonomy are essential for health," said the therapist and group leader Joann Peterson during our recent conversation on Gabriola Island. She is director of education at PD Seminars, a holistic healing and psychological growth centre. "We experience life through our bodies. If we are not able to articulate our life experience, our bodies speak what our minds and mouths cannot."

"A personal boundary," according to Dr. Peterson, "is an energetic experience of myself or the other person. I don't want to use the word *aura* because it is a new-age kind of word, but beyond where skin ends we have an energetic expression. We not only communicate boundaries verbally, but I think we have an energetic expression that is non-verbal." In her book *Anger, Boundaries, and Safety,* Dr. Peterson explains this concept in greater detail: "Boundaries are invisible, the result of a conscious, internal felt sense defining who I am. Asking yourself, 'In my life and relationships, what do I desire, want more of, or less of, or what don't I want, what are my stated limits?' begins the process. . . . In this self-definition, we define what we value and want in life at this particular time from a place of internal self-reference; *the locus of control is from inside ourselves.*"

Autonomy, then, is the development of that internal centre of control.

5. Attachment

Attachment is our connection with the world. In the earliest attachment relationships, we gain or lose the ability to stay open, self-nurturing and healthy. In those early attachment bonds, we learned to experience anger or to fear it and repress it. There we developed our sense of autonomy or suffered its atrophy. Connection is also vital to healing. Study after study concludes that people without social contact—the lonely ones—are at greatest risk for illness. People who enjoy genuine emotional support face a better prognosis, no matter what the disease.

Ever since a small nodule was found on his prostate fourteen years ago, seventy-one-year-old Derek has had annual PSA tests done. Two years ago he had a biopsy showing cancerous cells. "The oncologist said I was high risk, and he scared me. So I agreed to take six months of hormone therapy, which reduces the tumour. It kills your testosterone completely. You have to get a shot every three months. After the hormone treatment, the oncologist wanted to start radiation for seven weeks. I said no, I don't want this, because I've read so much about it. Radiation and surgery temporarily fix the problem, but after three to five years, it often comes back. And the radiation destroys so much . . . so many good cells in your body, besides the bad ones."

"What did you go through emotionally when you were diagnosed?"

"Well, you see, that has been the problem with me. I didn't tell anybody. I didn't tell any of my friends. I kept it all to myself, except for my wife and my two daughters.

"Before, I was a recluse. I was very private. Now, I'm very open. I love lots of people around me. Before, I didn't. I was perfectly happy to find a cave with a lock on the door, and I could live there happily for the rest of my life. My priorities have all changed. Before, I built steam locomotives for a hobby. I used to spend sixteen hours a day in my workshop doing that, and I was absolutely happy. Now, I haven't been in my workshop for two years, since I got cancer.

"Now, I need lots of people in my life. Cancer people support each other. And that's what we *need*—to talk about it. The rest of my life we will all be talking about it. It seems to be something that you have to do."

"Don't human beings in general need support and the opportunity to share emotions, and to talk about their difficulties, cancer or no cancer? Why do you think cancer would have to teach you this?"

"I wondered that myself. When I was first diagnosed, I built a wall around me, and I didn't let anybody in because I felt safe inside there. That was a mistake I made. I put all my energies into fighting the cancer, for eleven months. When I finally thought that the cancer was gone, I started to let this wall down, I started telling people about my experience, that I had cancer and that I had got rid of it. I was quite proud of the fact."

"You were able to share once you defeated the thing, but not while you were fighting it, when you most needed support. Why did you keep your wife out?"

"I never felt that she supported me . . . and yet . . . I know she was supporting me . . . but I wouldn't let her into my life. I had this wall around me, and I wouldn't let anybody in."

We sometimes find it easier to feel bitterness or rage than to allow ourselves to experience that aching desire for contact that, when disappointed, originally engendered the anger. Behind all our anger lies a deeply frustrated need for truly intimate contact. Healing both requires and implies regaining the vulnerability that made us shut down emotionally in the first place. We are no longer helplessly dependent children; we no longer need fear emotional vulnerability. We can permit ourselves to honour the universally reciprocal human need for connection and to challenge the ingrained belief that unconsciously burdens so many people with chronic illness: that we are not lovable. Seeking connections is a necessity for healing.

6. Assertion

Beyond acceptance and awareness, beyond the experience of anger and the unfolding of autonomy, along with the celebration of our capacity for attachment and the conscious search for contact, comes assertion: it is the declaration to ourselves and to the world that *we are* and that *we are who we are.*

Many times throughout this book we have witnessed people expressing the belief that if they do not act, they experience only emptiness, a frightening void. In our fear we falsely equate reality with tumult, being with activity, meaning with achievement. We think autonomy and freedom mean the liberty to do, to act or react as we wish. Assertion in the sense of self-declaration is deeper than the limited autonomy of action. It is the statement of our being, a positive valuation of ourselves independent of our history, personality, abilities or the world's perceptions of us. Assertion challenges the core belief that we must somehow justify our existence.

It demands neither acting nor reacting. It is *being,* irrespective of action.

Thus, assertion may be the very oppositive of action, not only in the narrow sense of refusing to do something we do not wish to do but *letting go of the very need to act.*

7. Affirmation

When we affirm, we make a positive statement; we move toward something of value. There are two basic values that can assist us to heal and to remain whole, if we honour them.

The first value is our own creative self. For many years after becoming a doctor, I was too caught up in my workaholism to pay attention to myself or to my deepest urges. In the rare moments I permitted any stillness, I noted a small fluttering at the pit of my belly, a barely perceptible disturbance. The faint whisper of a word would sound in my head: *writing*. At first I could not say whether it was heartburn or inspiration. The more I listened, the louder the message became: I needed to write, to express myself through written language not only so that others might hear me but so that I could hear myself.

The gods, we are taught, created humankind in their own image. Everyone has an urge to create. Its expression may flow through many channels: through writing, art or music, through the inventiveness of work or in any number of ways unique to all of us, whether it be cooking, gardening or the art of social discourse. The point is to honour the urge. To do so is healing for ourselves and for others; not to do so deadens our bodies and our spirits. When I did not write, I suffocated in silence.

"What is in us must out," wrote Hans Selye, "otherwise we may explode at the wrong places or become hopelessly hemmed in by frustrations. *The great art is to express our vitality through the particular channels and at the particular speed Nature foresaw for us.*"

The second great affirmation is of the universe itself—our connection with all that is. The assumption that we are cut off, alone and without contact is toxic, but—no matter how cruelly and how consistently life has shown us this dark shadow—it is no more than a bitter illusion. It forms part of the pathological biology of belief.

Physically it is easy to see that our sense of separateness from the universe is false: we do not go "from dust to dust," we are dust enlivened. We are a part of the universe with temporary consciousness, but never apart from it. Not by coincidence is the word *seeking* so frequently employed in relation to spiritual work.

Faced with illness, many people seek their spiritual selves almost instinctively, often in surprising ways. Anna, with breast cancer, was born Jewish and was brought up in her ancestral religion. She now goes to a Catholic cathedral for spiritual sustenance. "My beloved is God, and that's why I stay strong. I go to church, and I take Communion; I know that I am beloved of God. I serve at the altar. The first time I did it, I held the crucifix and two candles, and the priest said to me, 'You are the altar.' I've been saying that to myself, especially when I feel really awful: *I'm the altar.* And the priest said to me, 'If you're the altar of God there in the cathedral, you are the altar of God all the time. You are . . . beloved.'"

On the other hand, Lillian, a woman with arthritis I interviewed, has turned from Presbyterianism to Judaism. She grew up in a highly controlling and repressed home in her native Scotland. In her Jewish faith she finds a freedom to be herself, an acceptance and a joy of life long denied to her. She is still not quite liberated: when her brother comes to visit, she hides the menorah and the Sabbath candles. But she is more at peace than ever before. "I felt if I was going to heal, I would have to throw off spiritual bondage," she says.

Others I have spoken with have reaffirmed their confidence in their traditional faith, or they meditate, or they commune with nature. Each seeks his or her own way to the light within and without. For many it is not an easy search. No matter where we may have lost the key, like Nasruddin, we all prefer to begin under the street light where we can see.

"Seek and ye shall find," one of the great teachers said. The seeking itself is the finding, since one can fervently seek only what one already knows to exist.

Many people have done psychological work without ever opening to their own spiritual needs. Others have looked for healing only in the spiritual ways—in the search of God or universal Self—without ever realizing the importance of finding and developing the personal self. Health rests on three pillars: the body, the psyche and the spiritual connection. To ignore any one of them is to invite imbalance and dis-ease.

When it comes to healing, if we look only in the easy places, we usually find what Nasruddin and his neighbours found under the street light: *nothing.* Nasruddin, in his role as fool, did not know that. In his role as sage and teacher, he did.

Nasruddin, fool and sage, exists in all of us.

Notes

1: The Bermuda Triangle
1. Hans Selye, *The Stress of Life*, rev. ed. (New York: McGraw-Hill, 1978), 4.
2. M. Angell, "Disease as a Reflection of the Psyche," *New England Journal of Medicine*, 13 June 1985.
3. Interview with Dr. Robert Maunder.
4. Plato, *Charmides*, quoted in A. A. Brill, *Freud's Contribution to Psychiatry*, (New York, W. W. Norton, 1944), 233.

2: The Little Girl Too Good to Be True
1. G. M. Franklin, "Stress and Its Relationship to Acute Exacerbations in Multiple Sclerosis," *Journal of Neurological Rehabilitation* 2, no. 1 (1988).
2. I. Grant, "Psychosomatic-Somatopsychic Aspects of Multiple Sclerosis," in U. Halbriech, ed., *Multiple Sclerosis: A Neuropsychiatric Disorder*, no. 37, *Progress in Psychiatry* series (Washington/London: American Psychiatric Press).
3. V. Mei-Tal, "The Role of Psychological Process in a Somatic Disorder: Multiple Sclerosis," *Psychosomatic Medicine* 32, no. 1 (1970), 68.
4. G. S. Philippopoulous, "The Etiologic Significance of Emotional Factors in Onset and Exacerbations of Multiple Sclerosis," *Psychosomatic Medicine* 20 (1958): 458–74.
5. Mei-Tal, "The Role of Psychological Process . . . ," 73.
6. I. Grant, "Severely Threatening Events and Marked Life Difficulties Preceding Onset or Exacerbation of Multiple Sclerosis," *Journal of Neurology, Neurosurgery and Psychiatry* 52 (1989): 8–13. Seventy-seven per cent of the MS group, but only 35 per cent of the control group, experienced marked life adversity in the year prior to the appearance of disease. "The excess in marked life stress was most evident in the 6 months before onset. . . . 24 of 39 multiple sclerosis patients (62 per cent) reported a severely threatening event, as compared with six of 40 controls (15 per cent). . . . Significantly more patients than controls experienced marital difficulties (49 per cent vs. 10 per cent). . . . Eighteen of 23 first cases and 12 of 16 relapsing cases reported marked adversity."
7. J. D. Wilson., ed., *Harrison's Principles of Internal Medicine*, 12th ed. (New York: McGraw-Hill, 1999), 2039.
8. L. J. Rosner, *Multiple Sclerosis: New Hope and Practical Advice for People with MS and Their Families* (New York: Fireside Publishers, 1992), 15.
9. E. Chelmicka-Schorr and B. G. Arnason, "Nervous System–Immune System

Interactions and Their Role in Multiple Sclerosis," *Annals of Neurology,* supplement to vol. 36 (1994), S29–S32.

10. Elizabeth Wilson, *Jacqueline du Pré* (London: Faber and Faber, 1999), 160.

11. Hilary du Pré and Piers du Pré, *A Genius in the Family: An Intimate Memoir of Jacqueline du Pré* (New York: Vintage, 1998).

12. Wilson, *Jacqueline du Pré.*

3: Stress and Emotional Competence

1. Selye, *The Stress of Life,* xv.

2. Ibid., 414.

3. Ibid., 62.

4. Ibid., 150.

5. E. M. Sternberg (moderator), "The Stress Response and the Regulation of Inflammatory Disease," *Annals of Internal Medicine* 17, no. 10 (15 November 1992), 855.

6. A. Kusnecov and B. S. Rabin, "Stressor-Induced Alterations of Immune Function: Mechanisms and Issues," *International Archives of Allergy and Immunology* 105 (1994), 108.

7. Selye, *The Stress of Life,* 370.

8. S. Levine and H. Ursin, "What Is Stress?" in S. Levine and H. Ursin, eds., *Psychobiology of Stress* (New York: Academic Press), 17.

9. W. R. Malarkey, "Behavior: The Endocrine-Immune Interface and Health Outcomes," in T. Theorell, ed., *Everyday Biological Stress Mechanisms,* vol. 22, (Basel: Karger, 2001), 104–115.

10. M. A. Hofer, "Relationships as Regulators: A Psychobiologic Perspective on Bereavement," *Psychosomatic Medicine* 46, no. 3 (May–June 1984), 194.

11. Ross Buck, "Emotional Communication, Emotional Competence, and Physical Illness: A Developmental-Interactionist View," in J. Pennebaker and H. Treve, eds., *Emotional Expressiveness, Inhibition and Health* (Seattle: Hogrefe and Huber, 1993), 38.

12. Ibid.

4: Buried Alive

1. Suzannah Horgan, *Communication Issues and ALS: A Collaborative Exploration* (Thesis submitted to the Division of Applied Psychology, University of Alberta, Calgary, 2001).

2. Wolfgang J. Streit and Carol A. Kincaid-Colton, "The Brain's Immune System," *Scientific American* 273, no. 5 (November 1995).

3. W. A. Brown and P. S. Mueller, "Psychological Function in Individuals with Amyotrophic Lateral Sclerosis," *Psychosomatic Medicine* 32, no. 2 (March–April 1970), 141–52. The countervailing study is by J. L. Houpt *et al.,* "Psychological Characteristics of Patients with Amyotrophic Lateral Sclerosis," *Psychosomatic Medicine* 39, no. 5, 299–303.

4. A. J. Wilbourn and H. Mitsumoto, "Why Are Patients with ALS So Nice?" presented at the ninth International ALS Symposium on ALS/MND, Munich, 1998.

5: Ray Robinson, *Iron Horse: Lou Gehrig in His Time* (New York: W. W. Norton & Company, 1990).

6. Michael White and John Gribbin, *Stephen Hawking: A Life in Science* (London: Viking, 1992).

7. Dennis Kaye, *Laugh, I Thought I'd Die* (Toronto: Penguin Putnam, 1994).

8. Evelyn Bell, *Cries of the Silent* (Calgary: ALS Society of Alberta, 1999), 12.

9. Lisa Hobbs-Birnie, *Uncommon Will: The Death and Life of Sue Rodriguez* (Toronto: Macmillan Canada, 1994).

10. Jane Hawking, *Music to Move the Stars* (London: Pan/Macmillan, 1993).

11. Christiane Northrup, *Women's Bodies, Women's Wisdom: Creating Physical and Emotional Health and Healing* (New York: Bantam Books, 1998), 61.

5: Never Good Enough

1. Jill Graham *et al.*, "Stressful Life Experiences and Risk of Relapse of Breast Cancer: Observational Cohort Study," *British Medical Journal* 324 (15 June 2002).

2. D. E. Stewart *et al.*, "Attributions of Cause and Recurrence in Long-Term Breast Cancer Survivors," *Psycho-Oncology* (March–April 2001).

3. Sandra M. Levy and Beverly D. Wise, "Psychosocial Risk Factors and Disease Progression," in Cary L. Cooper, ed., *Stress and Breast Cancer* (New York: John Wiley & Sons, 1988), 77–96.

4. M. Wirsching, "Psychological Identification of Breast Cancer Patients Before Biopsy," *Journal of Psychosomatic Research* 26 (1982), cited in Cary L. Cooper, ed., *Stress and Breast Cancer* (New York: John Wiley & Sons, 1993), 13.

5. C. B. Bahnson, "Stress and Cancer: The State of the Art," *Psychosomatics* 22, no. 3 (March 1981), 213.

6: S. Greer and T. Morris, "Psychological Attributes of Women Who Develop Breast Cancer: A Controlled Study, *Journal of Psychosomatic Research* 19 (1975), 147–53.

7. C. L. Bacon *et al.* "A Psychosomatic Survey of Cancer of the Breast," *Psychosomatic Medicine* 14 (1952): 453–60, paraphrased in Bahnson, "Stress and Cancer."

8. Sandra M. Levy, *Behavior and Cancer* (San Francisco: Jossey-Bass, 1985), 166.

9. Betty Ford, *Betty: A Glad Awakening* (New York: Doubleday, 1987), 36.

6: You Are a Part of This Too, Mom

1. Betty Krawczyk, *Lock Me Up or Let Me Go* (Vancouver: Raincoast, 2002).

2. Betty Shiver Krawczyk, *Clayoquot: The Sound of My Heart* (Victoria: Orca Book Publishers, 1996).

7: Stress, Hormones, Repression and Cancer

1. D. M. Kissen and H. G. Eysenck, "Personality in Male Lung Cancer Patients," *Journal of Psychosomatic Research* 6 (1962), 123.

2. T. Cox and C. MacKay, "Psychosocial Factors and Psychophysiological Mechanisms in the Aetiology and Development of Cancers," *Social Science and Medicine* 16 (1982), 385.

3. R. Grossarth-Maticek *et al.*, "Psychosocial Factors as Strong Predictors of Mortality from Cancer, Ischaemic Heart Disease and Stroke: The Yugoslav Prospective Study," *Journal of Psychosomatic Research* 29, no. 2 (1985), 167–76.

4. C. B. Pert *et al.,* "Neuropeptides and Their Receptors: A Psychosomatic Network," *The Journal of Immunology* 135, no. 2 (August 1985).

5. Candace Pert, *Molecules of Emotion: Why You Feel the Way You Feel* (New York: Touchstone, 1999), 22–23.

6. E. R. De Kloet, "Corticosteroids, Stress, and Aging," *Annals of New York Academy of Sciences,* 663 (1992), 358.

7. Rajesh K. Naz, *Prostate: Basic and Clinical Aspects* (Boca Raton: CRC Press, 1997), 75.

8. J. K. Kiecolt-Glaser and R. Glaser, "Psychoneuroimmunology and Immunotoxicology: Implications for Carcinogenesis," *Psychosomatic Medicine* 61 (1999), 271–72.

9. C. Tournier *et al.*, "Requirement of JNK for Stress-Induced Activation of the Cytochrome c-Mediated Death Pathway," *Science* 288 (5 May 2000), 870–74.

10. W. Jung and M. Irwin, "Reduction of Natural Killer Cytotoxic Activity in Major Depression: Interaction between Depression and Cigarette Smoking," *Psychosomatic Medicine* 61 (1999), 263–70.

11. H. Anisman *et al.*, "Neuroimmune Mechanisms in Health and Disease: 2. Disease," *Canadian Medical Association Journal* 155, no. 8 (15 October 1996).

12. Levy, *Behavior and Cancer*, 146–47.

13. C. Shively *et al.*, "Behavior and Physiology of Social Stress and Depression in Female Cynomolgus Monkeys, *Biological Psychiatry* 41 (1997), 871–82.

14. M. D. Marcus *et al.*, "Psychological correlates of functional hypothalamic amenorrhea," *Fertility and Sterility* 76, no. 2 (August 2001), 315.

15. J. C. Prior, "Ovulatory Disturbances: They Do Matter," *Canadian Journal of Diagnosis*, February 1997.

16. J. G. Goldberg, ed., *Psychotherapeutic Treatment of Cancer Patients* (New York: The Free Press, 1981), 46.

17. B. A. Stoll, ed., *Prolonged Arrest of Cancer* (Chichester: John Wiley & Sons, 1982), 1.

18. Levy, *Behavior and Cancer*, 146.

19. C. L. Cooper, ed., *Stress and Breast Cancer* (Chichester: John Wiley & Sons, 1988), 32.

20. Ibid.

21. Ibid., 31–32.

22. Ibid., 123.

23. J. G. Goldberg, ed., *Psychotherapeutic Treatment of Cancer Patients*, 45.

24. L. Elit, "Familial Ovarian Cancer," *Canadian Family Physician* 47 (April 2001).

25. Gilda Radner, *It's Always Something* (New York: Simon and Schuster, 1989).

8: Something Good Comes Out of This

1. G. L. Lu-Yao *et al.*, "Effect of Age and Surgical Approach on Complications and Short-Term Mortality after Radical Prostatectomy—A Population-Based Study," *Urology* 54, no. 2 (August 1999), 301–7.

2. Larry Katzenstein, "Can the Prostate Test Be Hazardous to Your Health?" *The New York Times*, 17 February 1999.

3. Study discussed in the periodical *Cancer*, 1997, cited in ibid.

4. C. J. Newschaffer *et al.*, "Causes of Death in Elderly Cancer Patients and in a Comparison Nonprostate Cancer Cohort," *Journal of the National Cancer Institute* 92, no.8 (19 April 2000), 613–22.

5. *The Journal of the American Medical Association*, 5 May 1999.

6. S. M. Levy, ed., *Biological Mediators of Behavior and Disease: Neoplasia* (New York: Elsevier Biomedical, 1981), 76.

7. T. E. Seeman and B. S. McEwen, "Impact of Social Environment Characteristics on Neuroendocrine Regulation," *Psychosomatic Medicine* 58 (September–October 1996), 462.

8. D. France, "Testosterone, the Rogue Hormone, Is Getting a Makeover," *The New York Times*, 17 February 1999.

9. U. Schweiger *et al.*, "Testosterone, Gonadotropin, and Cortisol Secretion in Male Patients with Major Depression," *Psychosomatic Medicine* 61 (1999), 292–96.

10. Naz, *Prostate,* 14.

11. Roger S. Kirby *et al., Prostate Cancer* (St. Louis: Mosby, 2001), 29.

12. Ibid., 15.

13. Levy, *Biological Mediators . . .,* 74.

14. Naz, *Prostate,* 17.

15. Ibid., 87.

16. R. P. Greenberg and P. J. Dattore, "The Relationship between Dependency and the Development of Cancer," *Psychosomatic Medicine* 43, no. 1 (February 1981).

17. *New England Journal of Medicine* 340: 884–87, cited in *The Journal of the American Medical Association* (5 May 1999), 1575.

18. Andrew Kirtzman, *Rudy Giuliani: Emperor of the City* (New York: HarperPerennial, 2001).

19. Lance Armstrong, *It's Not about the Bike: My Journey Back to Life* (New York: Berkley Books, 2001).

20. A. Horwich, ed., *Testicular Cancer: Investigation and Management* (Philadelphia: Williams & Wilkins, 1991), 6.

9: Is There a "Cancer Personality"?

1. Levy, *Behavior and Cancer,* 19.

2: W. Kneier and L. Temoshok, "Repressive Coping Reactions in Patients with Malignant Melanoma as Compared to Cardiovascular Patients," *Journal of Psychosomatic Research* 28, no. 2 (1984), 145–55.

3. L. Temoshok and B. Fox, "Coping Styles and Other Psychosocial Factors Related to Medical Status and to Prognosis in Patients with Cutaneous Malignant Melanoma," in B. Fox and B. Newberry, eds., *Impact of Psychoendocrine Systems in Cancer and Immunity* (New York: C. J. Hogrefe, 1984), 263.

4. Levy, *Behavior and Cancer,* 17.

5. G. A. Kune *et al.,* "Personality as a Risk Factor in Large Bowel Cancer: Data from the Melbourne Colorectal Cancer Study," *Psychological Medicine* 21 (1991): 29–41.

6. C. B. Thomas and R. L. Greenstreet, "Psychobiological Characteristics in Youth as Predictors of Five Disease States: Suicide, Mental Illness, Hypertension, Coronary Heart Disease and Tumor," *Hopkins Medical Journal* 132 (January 1973), 38.

10: The 55 Per Cent Solution

1. Malcolm Champion *et al.,* eds., *Optimal Management of IBD: Role of the Primary Care Physician* (Toronto: The Medicine Group, 2001).

2. G. Moser *et al.,* "Inflammatory Bowel Disease: Patients' Beliefs about the Etiology of Their Disease—A Controlled Study," *Psychosomatic Medicine* 55 (1993), 131, cited in R. Maunder, "Mediators of Stress Effects in Inflammatory Bowel Disease: Not the Usual Suspects," *Journal of Psychosomatic Research* 48 (2000), 569–77.

3. G. L. Engel, as paraphrased in G. F. Solomon *et al.,* "Immunity, Emotions, and Stress," *Annals of Clinical Research* 6 (1974), 313–22.

4. G. L. Engel, "Studies of Ulcerative Colitis III: The Nature of the Psychological Process," *American Journal of Medicine* 19 (1955), 31, cited in A. Watkins, ed., *Mind-Body Medicine: A Clinician's Guide to Psychoneuroimmunology* (New York: Churchill Livingstone, 1997), 140.

5. D. A. Drossman, "Presidential Address: Gastrointestinal Illness and the Biopsychosocial Model," *Psychosomatic Medicine* 60 (1998): 258–67.

6. S. R.Targan, "Biology of Inflammation in Crohn's Disease: Mechanisms of Action of Anti-TNF-Alpha Therapy," *Canadian Journal of Gastroenterology: Update on Liver and Inflammatory Bowel Disease,* vol. 14, supplement C (September 2000).

7. H. Anisman *et al.,* "Neuroimmune Mechanisms in Health and Disease: 1: Health," *Canadian Medical Association Journal* 155, no. 7 (1 October 1996), 872.

8. Drossman, "Presidential Address," 265.

9. S. Levenstein *et al.,* "Stress and Exacerbation in Ulcerative Colitis: A Prospective Study of Patients Enrolled in Remission," *American Journal of Gastroenterology* 95, no. 5, 1213–20.

10. Noel Hershfield, "Hans Selye, Inflammatory Bowel Disease and the Placebo Response," *Canadian Journal of Gastroenterology* 11, no. 7 (October 1997): 623–24.

11: It's All in Her Head

1. Y. Ringel and D. A. Drossman, "Toward a Positive and Comprehensive Diagnosis of Irritable Bowel Syndrome," <*Medscape/gastro/journal*> 2, no. 6 (26 December 2000).

2. Drossman, "Presidential Address," 259.

3. Ibid.

4. E. A. Mayer and H. E. Raybould, "Role of Visceral Afferent Mechanisms in Functional Bowel Disorders," *Gastroenterology* 99 (December 1990): 1688–1704.

5. Drossman, "Presidential Address," 263.

6. Lin Chang, "The Emotional Brain, in Diagnosis and Management of Irritable Bowel Syndrome," (Oakville: Pulsus Group, 2001), 2. Highlights from a symposium held during Canadian Digestive Diseases Week, Banff, Alberta, 26 February 2001.

7. J. Lesserman *et al.,* "Sexual and Physical Abuse History in Gastroenterology Practice: How Types of Abuse Impact Health Status," *Psychosomatic Medicine* 58 (1996), 4–15.

8. Ibid.

9. M. D. Gershon, *The Second Brain: The Scientific Basis of Gut Instinct* (New York: HarperCollins, 1998), xiii.

10. Mayer and Raybould, "Role of Visceral Afferent Mechanisms in Functional Bowel Disorders."

11. Lin Chang, "The Emotional Brain . . ."

12. Drossman, "Presidential Address," 262.

13. L. A. Bradley *et al.,* "The Relationship between Stress and Symptoms of Gastroesophageal Reflux: The Influence of Psychological Factors," *American Journal of Gastroenterology* 88, no.1 (January 1993), 11–18.

14. W. J. Dodds *et al.,* "Mechanisms of Gastroesophageal Reflux in Patients with Reflux Esophagitis," *New England Journal of Medicine* 307, no. 25 (16 December 1982), 1547–52.

15. D. A. Drossman *et al.,* "Effects of Coping on Health Outcome among Women with Gastrointestinal Disorders," *Psychosomatic Medicine* 62 (2000), 309–17.

12: I Shall Die First from the Top

1. M. J. Meaney *et al.,* "Effect of Neonatal Handling on Age-Related Impairments Associated with the Hippocampus," *Science* 239 (12 February 1988), 766–68.

2. D. A. Snowdon *et al.,* "Linguistic Ability in Early Life and the Neuropathology of Alzheimer's Disease and Cerebrovascular Disease: Findings from the Nun Study," *Annals of the New York Academy of Sciences* 903 (April 2000), 34–38.

3. Victoria Glendinning, *Jonathan Swift: A Portrait* (Toronto: Doubleday Canada, 1998).

4. David Shenk, *The Forgetting: Alzheimer's: The Portrait of an Epidemic* (New York: Doubleday, 2001).

5. D. A. Snowdon, "Aging and Alzheimer's Disease: Lessons from the Nun Study," *Gerontologist* 38, no. 1 (February 1998), 5–6.

6. V. A. Evseev *et al.*, "Dysregulation in Neuroimmunopathology and Perspectives of Immunotherapy," *Bulletin of Experimental Biological Medicine* 131, no. 4 (April 2001), 305–308.

7. M. F. Frecker *et al.*, "Immunological Associations in Familial and Non-familial Alzheimer's Patients and Their Families," *Canadian Journal of Neurological Science* 21, no. 2 (May 1994), 112–19.

8. M. Popovic *et al.*, "Importance of Immunological and Inflammatory Processes in the Pathogenesis and Therapy of Alzheimer's Disease," *International Journal of Neuroscience* 9, no. 3–4 (September 1995), 203–36.

9. F. Marx *et al.*, "Mechanisms of Immune Regulation in Alzheimer's Disease: A Viewpoint," *Arch Immunol Ther Exp (Warsz)* 47, no. 4 (1999), 204–209.

10. J. K. Kiecolt-Glaser *et al.*, "Emotions, Morbidity, and Mortality: New Perspectives from Psychoneuroimmunology," *Annual Review of Psychology* 53 (2002), 83–107.

11. Edmund Morris, *Dutch: A Memoir of Ronald Reagan* (New York: Modern Library, 1999).

12. Michael Korda, *Another Life* (New York: Random House, 1999).

13: Self or Non-Self: The Immune System Confused

1. C. E. G. Robinson, "Emotional Factors and Rheumatoid Arthritis," *Canadian Medical Association Journal* 77 (15 August 1957), 344–45.

2. B. R. Shochet *et al.*, "A Medical-Psychiatric Study of Patients with Rheumatoid Arthritis," *Psychosomatics* 10, no. 5 (September–October 1969), 274.

3. John Bowlby, *Attachment,* 2nd ed. (New York: Basic Books, 1982), 377.

4. R. Otto and I. R. Mackay, "Psycho-Social and Emotional Disturbance in Systemic Lupus Erythematosus," *Medical Journal of Australia*, (9 September 1967), 488–93.

5. John Bowlby, *Loss* (New York: Basic Books, 1980), 69.

6. Bowlby, *Attachment,* 68.

7. Michael Hagmann, "A New Way to Keep Immune Cells in Check," *Science*, 1945.

8. P. Marrack and J. W. Kappler, "How the Immune System Recognizes the Body," *Scientific American*, September 1993.

9. G. F. Solomon and R. H. Moos, "The Relationship of Personality to the Presence of Rheumatoid Factor in Asymptomatic Relatives of Patients with Rheumatoid Arthritis," *Psychosomatic Medicine* 27, no. 4 (1965), 350–60.

10. M. W. Stewart *et al.*, "Differential Relationships between Stress and Disease Activity for Immunologically Distinct Subgroups of People with Rheumatoid Arthritis," *Journal of Abnormal Psychology* 103, no. 2 (May 1994), 251–58.

11. D. J. Wallace, "The Role of Stress and Trauma in Rheumatoid Arthritis and Systemic Lupus Erythematosus," *Seminars in Arthritis and Rheumatism* 16, no. 3 (February 1987), 153–57.

12. S. L. Feigenbaum *et al.*, "Prognosis in Rheumatoid Arthritis: A Longitudinal Study of Newly Diagnosed Adult Patients," *The American Journal of Medicine* 66 (March 1979).

13. J. M. Hoffman *et al.*, "An Examination of Individual Differences in the Relationship between Interpersonal Stress and Disease Activity Among Women with

Rheumatoid Arthritis," *Arthritis Care Research* 11, no. 4 (August 1998), 271–79.

14. J. M. Hoffman *et al.*, "Examination of Changes in Interpersonal Stress as a Factor in Disease Exacerbations among Women with Rheumatoid Arthritis," *Annals of Behavioral Medicine* 19, no. 3a (Summer 1997), 279–86.

15. L. R. Chapman, *et al.*, "Augmentation of the Inflammatory Reaction by Activity of the Central Nervous System," *American Medical Association Archives of Neurology* 1 (November 1959).

16. Hoffman, "Examination of Changes in Interpersonal Stress . . . "

14: A Fine Balance: The Biology of Relationships

1. Hofer, "Relationships as Regulators."

2. Buck, "Emotional Communication, Emotional Competence, and Physical Illness," 42.

3. Seeman and McEwen, "Impact of Social Environment Characteristics . . . "

4. E. Pennisi, "Neuroimmunology: Tracing Molecules That Make the Brain-Body Connection," *Science* 275 (14 February 1997), 930–31.

5. G. Affleck *et al.*, "Mood States Associated with Transitory Changes in Asthma Symptoms and Peak Expiratory Flow," *Psychosomatic Medicine* 62, 62–68.

6. D. A. Mrazek, "Childhood Asthma: The Interplay of Psychiatric and Physiological Factors," *Advances in Psychosomatic Medicine* 14 (1985), 16–32.

7. Ibid., 21.

8. I. Florin *et al.*, "Emotional Expressiveness, Psychophysiological Reactivity and Mother-Child Interaction with Asthmatic Children," in Pennebaker and Treve, *Emotional Expressiveness, Inhibition and Health*, 188–89.

9. S. Minuchin *et al*, "A Conceptual Model of Psychosomatic Illness in Children, Family Organization and Family Therapy," *Archives of General Psychiatry* 32 (August 1975), 1031–38.

10. M. A. Price *et al.*, "The Role of Psychosocial Factors in the Development of Breast Carcinoma. Part II: Life Event Stressors, Social Support, Defense Style, and Emotional Control and Their Interactions," *Cancer* 91, no. 4 (15 February 2001), 686–97.

11. P. Reynolds and G. A. Kaplan, "Social Connections and Risk for Cancer: Prospective Evidence from the Alameda County Study," *Behavioral Medicine*, (Fall 1990), 101–10.

12. For a full discussion of differentiation, see Michael E. Kerr and Murray Bowen, *Family Evaluation: An Approach Based on Bowen Theory* (New York: W. W. Norton & Company, 1988), chapter 4, 89–111.

13. S. E. Locke, "Stress, Adaptation, and Immunity: Studies in Humans," *General Hospital Psychiatry* 4 (1982), 49–58.

14. J. K. Kiecolt-Glaser *et al.*, "Marital Quality, Marital Disruption, and Immune Function," *Psychosomatic Medicine* 49, no. 1 (January–February 1987).

15. Kerr and Bowen, *Family Evaluation*, 182.

16. Seeman and McEwen, "Impact of Social Environment Characteristics . . .," 459.

15: The Biology of Loss

1. L. Grassi and S. Molinari, "Early Family Attitudes and Neoplastic Disease," Abstracts of the Fifth Symposium on Stress and Cancer, Kiev, 1984; cited in H. J. Baltrusch and M. E. Waltz, "Early Family Attitudes and the Stress Process—A Life-Span and Personological Model of Host-Tumor Relationships: Biopsychosocial Research on Cancer and Stress in Central Europe," in Stacey B. Day, ed., *Cancer, Stress and Death* (New York: Plenum Medical Book Company, 1986), 275.

2. Ibid., 277.

3. L. G. Russek et al., "Perceptions of Parental Caring Predict Health Status in Midlife: A 35-Year Follow-up of the Harvard Mastery Stress Study," *Psychosomatic Medicine* 59 (1997), 144–49.

4. M. A. Hofer, "On the Nature and Consequences of Early Loss," *Psychosomatic Medicine* 58 (1996), 570–80.

5. "Kisses and Chemistry Linked in Rats," *The Globe and Mail* (Toronto) 17 September 1997.

6. Hofer, "On the Nature and Consequences of Early Loss."

7. S. Levine and H. Ursin, "What is Stress?" in S. Levine and H. Ursin, eds., *Psychobiology of Stress*, (New York: Academic Press, 1972), 17.

8. Allan Schore, *Affect Regulation and the Origin of the Self: The Neurobiology of Emotional Development* (Mahwah: Lawrence Erlbaum Associates, 1994), 378.

16: The Dance of Generations

1. M. Marmot and E. Brunner, "Epidemiological Applications of Long-Term Stress in Daily Life," in T. Theorell, ed., *Everyday Biological Stress Mechanisms,* vol. 22 (Basel: Karger, 2001), 89–90.

2. C. Caldji et al., "Maternal Care During Infancy Regulates the Development of Neural Systems Mediating the Expression of Fearfulness in the Rat," *Neurobiology* 95, no. 9 (28 April 1998), 5335–40.

3. C. Caldji et al., "Variations in Maternal Care in Infancy Regulate the Development of Stress Reactivity," *Biological Psychiatry* 48, no. 12, 1164–74.

4. L. Miller et al., "Intergenerational Transmission of Parental Bonding among Women," *Journal of the American Academy of Child and Adolescent Psychiatry* 36 (1997), 1134–39.

5. R. Yehuda et al., "Cortisol Levels in Adult Offspring of Holocaust Survivors: Relation to PTSD Symptom Severity in the Parent and Child," *Psychoneuroendocrinology* 27, no. 1–2 (2001), 171–80.

6. D. J. Siegel, *The Developing Mind: Toward a Neurobiology of Interpersonal Experience* (New York: The Guilford Press, 1999), 73.

7. Selye, *The Stress of Life*, 81.

8. Kerr and Bowen, *Family Evaluation,* 259.

9. Caldji, "Variations In Maternal Care in Infancy . . ."

10. M. Kerr, "Cancer and the Family Emotional System," in J. G. Goldberg, ed., *Psychotherapeutic Treatment of Cancer Patients* (New York: The Free Press, 1981), 297.

11. Selye, *The Stress of Life*, 391.

12. D. Raphael, *Social Justice Is Good for Our Hearts: Why Societal Factors—Not Lifestyles—Are Major Causes of Heart Disease in Canada and Elsewhere* (Toronto: CSJ Foundation for Research and Education, 2002), xi; report available at http://www.socialjustice.org.

13. M. G. Marmot et al., "Inequalities in Death—Specific Explanations of a General Pattern," *Lancet* 3 (1984), 1003–6, cited in M. Marmot and E. Brunner, "Epidemiological Applications of Long-Term Stress in Daily Life," in T. Theorell, ed., *Everyday Biological Stress Mechanisms*, 83.

17: The Biology of Belief
1. B. H. Lipton, "Nature, Nurture and Human Development," *Journal of Prenatal and Perinatal Psychology and Health* 16, no. 2 (2001), 167–80.

18: The Power of Negative Thinking
1. Kerr and Bowen, *Family Evaluation*, 279.
2. Mogens R. Jensen, "Psychobiological Factors Predicting the Course of Breast Cancer," *Journal of Personality* 55, no. 2 (June 1987), 337.
3. Levy, *Behavior and Cancer*, 165.
4. S. Warren *et al.*, "Emotional Stress and the Development of Multiple Sclerosis: Case-Control Evidence of a Relationship," *Journal of Chronic Disease* 35 (1982), 821–31.
5. Ford, *A Glad Awakening*.
6. Candace B. Pert, *Molecules of Emotion,* 193.

19: The Seven A's of Healing
1. A. J. Bdurtha *et al.*, "A Clinical, Histologic, and Immunologic Study of a Case of Metastatic Malignant Melanoma Undergoing Spontaneous Remission," *Cancer* 37 (1976), 735–42.
2. Rogentine *et al.*, cited in B. Fox and B. Newberry, eds., *Impact of Psychoendocrine Systems in Cancer and Immunity* (New York: C. J. Hogrefe, 1984), 259.
3. Ibid., 267.
4. F. I. Fawzy *et al.*, "Malignant Melanoma: Effects of an Early Structured Psychiatric Intervention, Coping, and Affective State on Recurrence and Survival 6 Years Later," *Archives of General Psychiatry* 50 (1993), 681–89; cited in Michael Lerner, *Choices in Healing* (Cambridge, Mass.: The MIT Press, 1994), 159.
5. F. I. Fawzy *et al.*, "A Structured Psychiatric Intervention for Cancer Patients: Changes over Time in Immunologic Measures," *Archives of General Psychiatry* 47 (1990), 729–35.
6. Oliver Sacks, *The Man Who Mistook His Wife for a Hat and Other Clinical Tales* (New York: HarperPerennial, 1990).
7. A. F. Siegman *et al.*, "Antagonistic Behavior, Dominance, Hostility, and Coronary Heart Disease," *Psychosomatic Medicine* 62 (2000), 248–57.
8. L. R. Ormont, "Aggression and Cancer in Group Treatment" in Jane G. Goldberg, ed., *The Psychotherapy of Cancer Patients* (New York: The Free Press, 1981), 226.
9. V. J. Felitti *et al.*, "Relationship of Childhood Abuse and Household Dysfunction to Many of the Leading Causes of Death in Adults: The Adverse Childhood Experiences (ACE) Study," *American Journal of Preventative Medicine* 14, no. 4 (1998), 245–58.

Resources

THE FOLLOWING IS A SHORT list of resources for people interested in healing, or in preventing ill health. It focuses on programs that deal with understanding and reducing stress or with identifying and releasing the grip of the ingrained biology of belief. Not included here are the many local and national support groups for specific conditions such as multiple sclerosis, ALS, arthritis, fibromyalgia, chronic fatigue, breast cancer, ovarian cancer and so on.

1. Beginning Your Healing Journey: An Active Response to the Crisis of Cancer
A program developed by Dr. Alastair J. Cunningham, himself a cancer survivor. He is Professor of Medical Biophysics and Psychiatry at the University of Toronto, and is a world renowned researcher in psycho-oncology. He holds Ph.D. degrees in cell biology and psychology and has lectured extensively in the United States, Canada, Europe, Australia and New Zealand on his research on healing and his findings. *The Healing Journey* is based on Dr. Cunningham's work with cancer patients at the Ontario Cancer Institute over twenty years. His approach includes an exploration of what stress is, relaxation, guided mental imagery, thought management and other techniques.

Dr. Cunningham's research has shown "a strong association between longer survival . . .related to the involvement of cancer patients in psychological self-help activities." Although he has worked extensively with cancer, I have no doubt that his techniques would help people with any of the conditions discussed in *When the Body Says No. The Healing Journey* is available internationally in a series of videotapes, audiotapes and a book. It may be purchased from the non-profit World Health Services Council, whose toll-free phone number is 1-866-999-9909. Web site: http://www.beginningyourhealingjourney.org.

2. The Canadian Institute of Stress
Founded in 1979 by Dr. Hans Selye, the CIS runs educational programs on stress for institutions and companies, provides speakers, and offers stress assessment and counselling for individuals. Tele-classes are also available, conducted by telephone. The director of the CIS is Dr. Richard Earle, formerly a close colleague of Dr. Selye's at McGill University. Canadian

Institute of Stress, Medcan Clinic Office, Suite 1500, 150 York Street, Toronto, Ontario, Canada M5H 3S5. Phone: (416) 236–4218. Web site: http://www.stresscanada.org.

3. The Health News Network

An online resource centre for the study of body and mind in health and illness, stress management and disease prevention. Available here are capsule discussions of many of the issues covered in *When the Body Says No* and a long list of links for particular diseases and conditions. Web site: http://www.healthnewsnet.com.

4. The Landmark Forum

The Landmark Forum is a program available in many countries, run by the Landmark Education Corporation. I have participated in it personally. The Landmark Forum is the single most powerful program I know of for dissolving the entrenched biology of belief. Their technique works to help people get into the present by completing the past—that is, to let go of imperatives, perceptions and motivations derived from our early interpretations of childhood experience. As shown throughout this book, it is these fixed but unconcious interpretations that underlie and trigger many of our chronic stresses. The initial Landmark event is a three-day workshop, followed by a weekly evening seminar. I warmly recommend it for people at any stage of life as an essential educational and transformative experience in reducing and eliminating the self-imposed stresses I have written about in this book. Web site: http://www.landmarkeducation.com.

5. pd Seminars, Gabriola Island, British Columbia

Based on Gabriola Island, British Columbia, pd Seminars is an organization devoted to personal growth and healing. It was founded by two physicians, Bennet Wong and Jock McKeen, who felt a need to expand their understanding of health beyond the traditional Western model. The residential programs for personal and professional development run by pd Seminars vary in duration from a few days to several weeks and offer a broad array of approaches—from meditation, thought-field therapy, music, writing and movement, to anger expression, the learning of boundaries, energetics and breath training. Many people with chronic illness or chronic stress have benefited from one or more of the pd programs. Phone: (250) 247–9211 Web site: http://www.pdseminars.com.

6. Dr. Bruce Lipton

The work of molecular biologist Dr. Bruce Lipton has helped bridge the gap between basic sciences and developmental psychology. Formerly Associate Professor of Anatomy at the University of Wisconsin School of Medicine, Dr. Lipton has shown how the biology of belief is ingrained at the very cellular level. He is also developing techniques to help people free themselves from that early psycho-biological programming. Information regarding his dynamic video lectures is available at his Web site: http://www.brucelipton.com.

Acknowledgments

OWE A GREAT DEBT OF gratitude to the many people, some of them former patients and some newly met, who open-heartedly shared their life histories, their sufferings and their souls so that others may possibly learn by reading what they have had to learn through painful experience.

Diane Martin at Knopf Canada supported this work since it was no more than a few words over dinner, four years ago. She slogged through a painfully long manuscript with interest and with compassion for author and reader, both of whom have benefited from her professionally astute guidance. I am also grateful to Tom Miller of John Wiley & Sons in New York, who recognized the possibilities of my book proposal where other U.S. publishers could see only "yet another book on stress."

Ceara O'Mara Sullivan in Virginia was my heaven-sent unofficial critic/editor/co-writer and long-distance friend. She dropped in unannounced via the Internet, serendipitously, and proceeded, expertly, to make the writing of the book—if not always my life—a lot easier. This volume would not be in front of the reader in its present form without her help.

My agent, Denise Bukowski, has ensured that *When the Body Says No* will be published in at least five countries and several languages and, beyond that, gave me editorial advice at a very late stage that transformed the manuscript into something much closer to what I had originally intended.

Heather Dundass and Elsa Deluca provided indispensable technical assistance in faithfully transcribing over two hundred hours of interviews.

My wife and soul-partner, Rae, has been a rigorous critic and a devoted and insightful supporter. Much that should not be in this book has been deleted thanks to her emotional courage, love and wisdom. Much that I cherish is present in my life owing to the very same qualities.

Grateful acknowledgment is made to the following for permission to reprint previously published material. Every reasonable effort has been made to contact copyright holders; in the event
of an inadvertent omission or error, please notify the publisher.

ALS Society of Alberta: Excerpt from *Cries of the Silent.* Copyright © ALS Society of Alberta
1999. 400-23 Ave. SW, Calgary, AB, T25 0J2.

Bantam Books, a division of Random House, Inc.: Excerpt from *Women's Bodies, Women's Wisdom*
by Christiane Northrup, M.D.

Berkley Books: Excerpt from *It's Not About the Bike: My Journey Back to Life* by Lance Armstrong.
Reprinted by permission of Berkley Books, a division of Penguin Putnam.

International Creative Management Inc. Excerpt from *It's Always Something.* Reprinted by permission of International Creative Management Inc. Copyright © 1989 by Gilda Radner. *Simon &*
Schuster, Inc.: Excerpt from *It's Always Something.* Reprinted with the permission of Simon &
Schuster, Inc., from *It's Always Something* by Gilda Radner, copyright © 1989 by Gilda Radner,
copyright © renewed 1990 by The Estate of Gilda Radner.

McGraw-Hill Education: Excerpt from *The Stress of Life.* Copyright © 1978 by Hans Selye.
Reproduced with permission of The McGraw Hill Companies.

Orca Book Publishers: Excerpt from *Clayoquot: Sound of My Heart* by Betty Krawczyk. Published
by Orca Book Publishers, Victoria, BC.

Pan MacMillan: Excerpt from *Music to Move the Stars* by Jane Hawking. Reprinted by permission
of MacMillan, London, UK.

Raincoast Books: Excerpt from *Lock Me Up or Let Me Go.* Published in 2002 by Press Gang, an
imprint of Raincoast Books. Text © 2002 by Betty Krawczyk.

Random House, Inc.: Excerpt from *Dutch* by Edmund Morris.

Random House, Inc.: Excerpt from *Another Life* by Michael Korda.

Random House of Canada, Ltd.: Excerpt from *Since You Asked.* Copyright © 1998 by Pamela
Wallin. Reprinted by permission of Random House Canada.

Simon & Schuster, Inc.: Excerpt from *Molecules of Emotion.* Reprinted with permission of Scribner,
a Division of Simon & Schuster from *Molecules of Emotion* by Candace B. Pert. Copyright ©
1997 by Candace B. Pert.

Simon & Schuster, Inc.: Excerpt from *The Man Who Mistook His Wife for a Hat and Other Clinical*
Tales. Reprinted with the permission of Simon & Schuster, Inc. from *The Man Who Mistook His*
Wife for a Hat and Other Clinical Tales by Oliver Sacks. Copyright © 1970, 1981, 1983, 1984, 1985
by Oliver Sacks.

Sterling Lord Literistic, Inc.: Excerpt from *Rudy Giuliani: Emperor of New York.* Reprinted by permission of Sterling Lord Literistic, Inc. Copyright Andrew Kirtzman.

W. W. Norton & Company, Inc.: Excerpt from *Iron Horse: Lou Gehrig in His Time,* by Ray Robinson.

Index

Gabor Maté, M.D., is a physician, public speaker, and award-winning author who lives in Vancouver, British Columbia. His most recent book, *In the Realm of Hungry Ghosts: Close Encounters with Addiction*, expresses his groundbreaking perspective on addictions; his unique take on ADD is found in his first book, *Scattered*. This work on the mind-body unity, *When the Body Says No,* has been published in over twelve languages on five continents. For more information, visit www.drgabormate.com.